RVUs

Applications for Medical Practice Success

3RD Edition

Frank D. Cohen, MBB, MPA

MGMA-ACMPE
104 Inverness Terrace East
Englewood, CO 80112-5306
877.275.6462
mgma.com

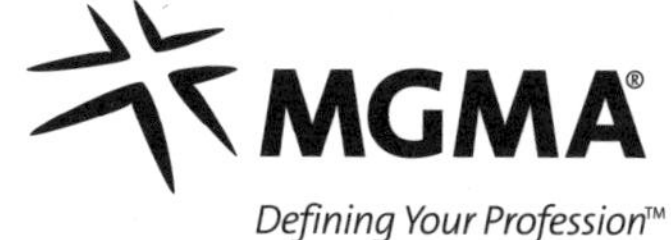

Medical Group Management Association® (MGMA®) publications are intended to provide current and accurate information and are designed to assist readers in becoming more familiar with the subject matter covered. Such publications are distributed with the understanding that MGMA does not render any legal, accounting, or other professional advice that may be construed as specifically applicable to individual situations. No representations or warranties are made concerning the application of legal or other principles discussed by the authors to any specific factual situation, nor is any prediction made concerning how any particular judge, government official, or other person will interpret or apply such principles. Specific factual situations should be discussed with professional advisors.

Production Credits
Acquisitions Editor: Susan L. Sarapata
Subject Matter Expert Reviewer: Laura Palmer
Editorial Reviewer: Judith H. Lento, BSH, CMPE
Editorial/Production Project Manager: Mary Kay Kozyra
Compositor: Virginia Howe
Proofreader: Carol Smith
Indexer: Sara Lynn Easter

Library of Congress Cataloging-in-Publication Data
Cohen, Frank.
RVUs : applications for medical practice success / Frank D. Cohen. -- 3rd ed.
p. ; cm.
Rev. ed. of: RVUs : applications for medical practice success / Kathryn P. Glass. 2nd ed. 2008.
Includes bibliographical references and index.
ISBN 978-1-56829-396-7
I. Glass, Kathryn P. RVUs. II. Medical Group Management Association. III. American College of Medical Practice Executives. IV. Title.
[DNLM: 1. Relative Value Scales--United States. 2. Fees, Medical--United States. 3. Practice Management, Medical--economics--United States. W 74 AA1]
R728
610.68'1--dc23
2013004841

Item
ISBN: 978-1-56829-396-7

Printed in the United States of America
10 9 8 7 6 5 4 3 2 1

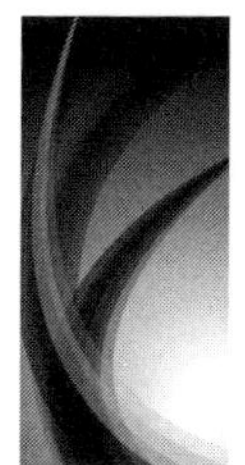

Contents

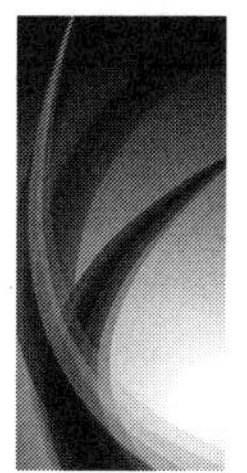

List of Exhibits

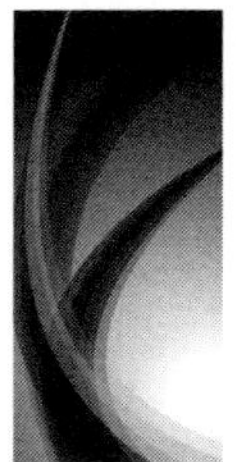

Preface

Back in 1990 I was preparing for a "new and improved" payer model for physicians under the Medicare program. At that time, the Health Care Financing Administration was in the testing phases for what we now know as the RBRVS, or resource-based relative value scale. It was hardly resource based and definitely not a relational model, at least not at that time. Upon its arrival in 1992, it received much less fanfare than I had expected. This may have been due to the introduction of the new evaluation and management (E/M) codes that were tied to the RBRVS in that they were designed to quantify the resources expended by a provider during a patient encounter. In those early days between release and adaption, I worked with my friends Steve Arter and Dennis Flint to create a national seminar series on RBRVS. The purpose of the series was to educate the masses on what was to become the standard in our industry for much more than it had initially been intended. Steve and I met by happenstance but soon formed an alliance that was steeped in physician advocacy, a friendship that remains to this day. The idea was simple — design an educational program that would bring physicians and their staff up to speed on the new payer model. But there's a big difference between simple and easy, and easy it was not! We had two weeks to accomplish the task, and Dennis (Flintstone, as I soon came to call him) and I locked ourselves in a small office and worked around the clock to produce our several-hundred-page manual (and interpretation) of what RBRVS meant both technically and operationally.

The coming of the MAAC system (maximum actual allowed payment), which was a quasi-fee-for-service model, and RBRVS posed many challenges. Perhaps the greatest was that it was likely released too early, that is, before it was ready for prime time. In the world according to Frank (the author of this book), which you are welcome to disregard, RBRVS was in its beta stages all the way through 1996. This period included significant changes to the practice expense methodologies, the use of more than one conversion factor, disagreements on how the new E/M codes (which, by the way, accounted for nearly a quarter of all codes submitted to Medicare) correlated with the real value they were assigned, and the beginning of a political battle that was preceded by the Gramm–Rudman–Hollings Balanced Budget Act of 1985. The latter evolved into the Medicare Balanced Budget Act of 1997 and was later followed by the Medicare sustainable growth rate formula (or better yet, debacle) that has, to this day, been a headache for physicians and should stand as an embarrassment to the Department of Health and Human Services.

Add to the above that RBRVS is now, for the most part, designed around the five-year updates from the Relative Value Scale Update Committee. This committee uses a very controversial method known as a RASCH estimate, and I remained unsurprised that just the mention of RBRVS invokes anger and controversy among many physicians and physician organizations. Anesthesiologists separated themselves from the existing methodology early in the game, and the jury is still out as to whether this was a benefit or not. Rumor has it that the American Academy of Neurology has considered developing an alternative to the RBRVS. And as admirable as this may be, it seems akin to the probability that Texas will really secede from the union anytime soon.

To some, RBRVS is a blessing. Aside from the fact that it was initially designed for Medicare as a payment model, there were other obvious opportunities that it offered from a business perspective. Some of these benefits would not be realized until later, after it evolved from its initial national beta test to something that was workable. The possibilities for developing private fee schedules were perhaps the first non-Medicare uses. To others, RBRVS is a curse, nothing more than a tool that the government uses to manipulate physicians and the services they provide and one that payers use to ensure that they don't have to pay physicians a reasonable amount for providing quality care to their patients.

Unfortunately, private payers saw the opportunity to use RBRVS to further suppress payments to providers while recognizing their opportunistic tendencies. Many were concerned; few were surprised. Internally, some practices and consultants recognized that if, in fact, this new system was resource based, then it might be a better way to develop cost analyses that were tied more closely to products and services. This was similar to what

Lean Accounting was about in those days. And if it could be tied to cost accounting, then it could be applied in a number of important administrative and operational ways. Global analyses would later resolve to more granular levels, such as estimating costs for any given procedure. This, used smartly, could have empowered physicians to more effectively negotiate rates with payers. But alas, the "could have" was dependent upon practices that actually adopted business intelligence, which was a premature assumption, at least early on. There was a period in the late 1990s when this idea caught on. Physicians began to recognize that they could isolate code groups into profit centers by either negotiating for better rates or dropping some procedures and/or services altogether. It appeared that physicians were finally recognizing their role as businessmen and businesswomen and the impact that performing like a business could have on the industry as a whole. However, that faded and we somehow took two steps backward. In the last few years, the industry has looked a lot like it did in the mid-1980s when hospitals went on spending sprees with the goal of "purchasing" as many physicians as possible. This may have taken the steam out of the engine. Physicians, now losing their autonomy, were becoming employees with less and less say and less and less concern over how the business model was treated. More recently, and closer to home, insurance companies are purchasing medical practices, as happened to my own physician's practice in Largo, Florida, only a few months ago.

None of this has gone unnoticed nor has every provider shied away from what has been a significant advance in the business technology of our industry. In 1999, I wrote a book on reengineering the way in which medical practices are managed. In that same year, perhaps the greatest pioneer in our industry advocating for change in the way we do business, Dr. Jeffrey Rose, now chief medical information officer with the Trizetto Group, LLC, wrote a book titled Medicine and the Information Age. Not to go unmentioned, Dr. Julie Silver published a book titled The Business of Medicine, which I thought should have inspired many other physicians to look at ways to improve not only our jobs but our industry.

So here we are some 20 years after the release of RBRVS and we are still battling over the methodology, applications, value, and appropriateness of RBRVS in the medical practice. Here's the sad part: it's like a summer-camp crush; time to get over it. Like it or hate it, RBRVS is here and it will likely play a major role in how physicians are paid in the future. So . . . get over it and get on with it. I salute those who think they can find a way to change it, but my advice is this—find another job. In this book, my goal is not to get you to like RBRVS but rather to teach you how to use it in such a way as to provide value and benefits to your organization. You can hate it, if you like, but don't ignore it. As members of the St. Petersburg Mad Dogs Triathlon Club like to say, "If you can't run with the big dogs, stay on the porch and don't bark."

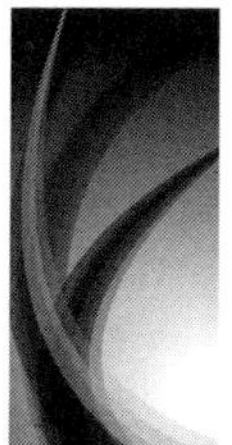

CHAPTER 1

Understanding Information Technology

Integrating the concepts of information technology into the medical practice, although a giant step toward converting to a business model, is only the first step in this paradigm shift.

WHAT IS INFORMATION TECHNOLOGY?

Depending on the industry to which one is connected, information technology (IT) can mean a lot of different things. In data management, for example, it may refer to accessing and managing large databases on a company's customers, products, or purchasing patterns. In telecommunications, it may represent data streams, switching information systems, or frequency tracking. In the computer field, it often refers to the integration of hardware and network systems with operating systems and expert applications.

In any case, no matter the industry, IT always refers to the management of the information necessary to strategically accomplish a given task or goal based upon the data available. Healthcare is no different. IT is about managing the massive amount of data now available in this industry in order to move ahead with strategic planning and the prospect of marking your territory as you go.

Depending on the industry, information technology can have many different meanings. In any case, it is the science of managing large amounts of information.

HOW IS INFORMATION TECHNOLOGY USED IN THE MEDICAL PRACTICE?

There are four basic areas of IT that are applicable to the medical practice with respect to the integration of business models, as follows:

- *Data mining* is a relatively new area for healthcare, particularly as it pertains to predictive analytics. Data mining is what Amazon.com

With respect to healthcare, there are four major uses for information technology:

- *Data mining*
- *Benchmarking*
- *Remediation*
- *Referential*

uses to understand who their customers are and the types of products they purchase. Pandora.com uses data mining and predictive analytics to recommend new songs to existing customers. In healthcare, the Centers for Medicare & Medicaid Services is now using data mining to identify error-prone providers and is using predictive analytics to predict the likelihood that a particular claim may be fraudulent or billed in error.

- *Benchmarking* is a method that is used to develop a standard by which other metrics can be compared. You may use benchmarking to develop a baseline evaluation and management utilization study and then compare it to your data set six months down the road using the same methodology. Or you may establish a cost accounting model, make some changes, and then measure your cost per relative value unit again in several months to measure your progress (or lack of progress, as the case may be).
- *Remediation* is a process whereby problems are identified and changes made immediately. This is more in the line with process improvement than with reengineering. However, after any reengineering project, process improvement becomes an integral component of regular business maintenance. Remediation would occur in a fee analysis, for example, if the practice were to identify fees that were below a minimum threshold or above a maximum threshold. The fees for those procedures would be immediately changed and implemented into the existing fee schedule.
- *Referential* models are used almost exclusively for information purposes. For example, a procedure code analysis could provide a reference model for coding and billing in a user-friendly format so that the coders and billers could actually use the information provided. You might see this commonly used as a filtered report of the Correct Coding Initiative edits, limited by the actual procedure codes used within a specific practice.

In the past, the practice did not have access to enough information. Today, there is too much information available, and many people don't know how to manage it to their benefit.

WHERE DID INFORMATION TECHNOLOGY START?

In the past, you didn't have enough information to effectively plan and track your business efforts. In the 1980s, when the health insurance industry began integrating commercial business techniques into their daily management processes, they brought with them the ability to produce and manage large amounts of data. For the most part, the focus in the healthcare industry was changed from patient care to financial modeling, at least from the perspective of the payers. At that time, there were no perceived problems within the industry because the patient cycle, including coding and billing, was pretty simple and industry regulation was almost nonexistent.

The problem many practices face today is that there is too much information for them to manage. Not all information is useful; not all information is valuable; and not all information is accurate or readily accessible. In order to manage the large amount of existing data in a cost-effective and efficient manner, one has to be able to understand and use relational software and understand the concept of interactive database management systems. Within the past 10 years, as a direct result of the Internet and an increase in the power of desktop computers, providers have gained access to the same data that are available to the payer side. Also, providers have the same ability to collect, process, analyze, and use that data to their advantage.

In the past, nobody in healthcare integrated information technology concepts into the practice of medicine.

In Exhibit 1.1, you can see that in the mid-1980s, the private sector (third-party and commercial insurers) was about 60 percent vested in integrating new nonclinical business and IT into their organizations. At the same time, the medical practice was only about 15 percent integrated with respect to the same methodology. The healthcare consultant, more inclined to mirror the medical practice, may have been 20 percent integrated, at the very most. The majority of consultants, however, were either equal to or slightly behind the practice.

In Exhibit 1.2, you can see that the insurance industry continued to move toward a fully integrated business model, while the medical practice remained relatively stagnant in this regard. Healthcare consultants, not sure of where the trend was heading, were hesitant to invest much time, capital, and other resources to move farther away from the medical practice for fear of missing the mark or alienating clients.

When the payer side realized the financial benefit of applying information technology concepts to the insurance sector, integration became an important part of payer strategic plans.

EXHIBIT 1.1 Integration of Information Technology, 1975–1985

0	10	20	30	40	50	60	70	80	90	100
	Medical Practice	Consultants				Payers				

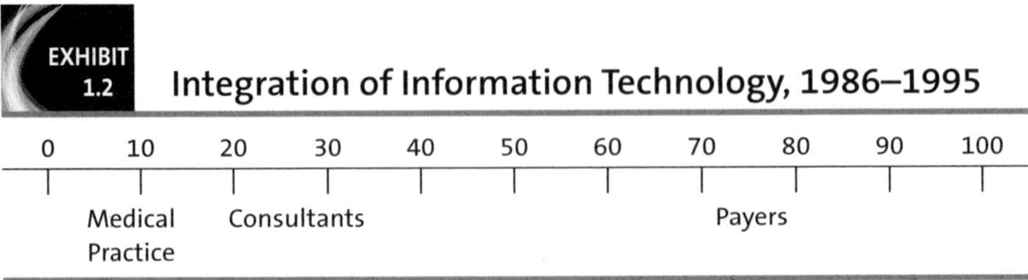

EXHIBIT 1.2 Integration of Information Technology, 1986–1995

One problem centered on the consultants' inability to adapt to the massive changes relating to both the financial markets and the regulatory industries. Many had grown along with the medical practice, getting their cues from the provider side, not the payer side. This limited, to a great degree, the trending that was necessary to keep up with the changes. Because the private sector has been very dynamic in this trending toward business integration, getting even a little behind the curve at the beginning can cause a logjam in experiential ways. This is similar to what happens when even one car slows for a few seconds on a busy highway.

Another problem was that many of the generalists lacked either the formal training or experience necessary to internalize the new technology being introduced, particularly in the area of IT. There were few programs available to teach this discipline. Specialty consultants, such as IT experts, process engineers, lawyers, accountants, coders, compliance officers, and quality control professionals, were seeing their business increase significantly. At the same time, the generalist was being remanded to the ranks of "referralists."

It is interesting to note that this trend closely mirrors the process of going through the provider system for a complex health condition. First, one must see the primary care physician to get an overall assessment of the condition. Then, if the generalist cannot handle the problem or feels that the patient should see a specialist, a referral is made. Depending upon the payment classification (i.e., fee-for-service, capitation, etc.), the generalist

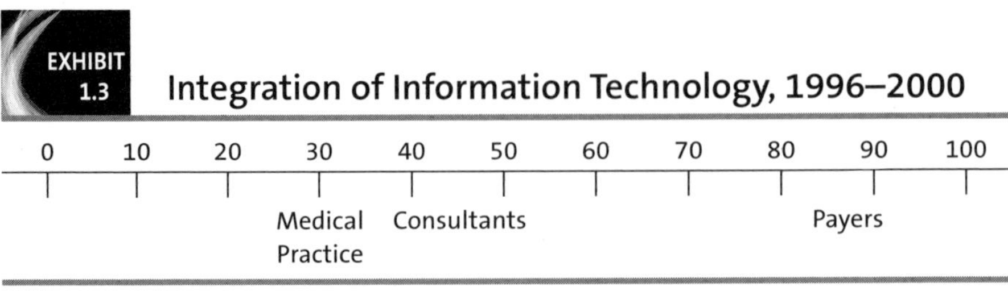

EXHIBIT 1.3 Integration of Information Technology, 1996–2000

may be more or less motivated to refer the patient as opposed to getting paid (or reducing transfer of revenue) for the service him- or herself. This has always posed a question of quality control and patient outcome.

By the year 2000, most payers had become, for the most part, integrated, while medical practices and consultants remained behind the eight ball.

Exhibit 1.3 illustrates the aggressive manner in which the insurance industry chose to embrace and move ahead toward total integration. The medical practice predictably remained far behind the move. However, there was a more aggressive move on the consultant side toward specialization and multidisciplinary team models, a type of vertical integration. Part of this was due to the difficulty, if not impossibility, of one consultant becoming expert in enough areas to satisfy all of the practices' needs. The generalist, still around but flailing for a purpose, was near the lower end of the vertical integration scale. The specialist, while not much farther ahead, was able to simulate integration because of the team model.

Again, this consultant model very closely mirrored the types of medical practice models being developed on the provider side. In order to deal effectively with managed care contracts and declining payment as a result of capitation, discounted fees, and other types of payment policies, medical practices formed many different types of organizations. All were geared toward building vertical integration into the clinical treatment side of their businesses. Certainly there were benefits of size, hence leverage, that allowed them to negotiate more effectively. The greatest benefit came, however, in their use of this integrated business model to develop a foundational base of good data and information that was used to determine profitability from all sides. Using IT as a tool, they were able to look at their practices from the same perspective as the payers. They knew going in, for example, whether a potential contract was profitable, eliminating the costs involved in having it reviewed by an attorney if it was not. The formation of these models, such as the Independent Practice Association (IPA), allowed the providers to loosely organize for the benefit of cross-referral while at the same time allowing them an arm's-length relationship to pursue their own practice interests.

In looking at the progressive development in healthcare consulting, there was, in effect, the same trend. Instead of an IPA, it is referred to as an ICA, or independent consultant association. Here you have generalists who provide the cursory review of the practice's problem, resolving those issues that are within their area of expertise and base of experience and training. Situations that require specialized care are referred to the appropriate specialists. This team approach model, or vertical integration of specialties, is still driven by a primary care foundation, hence the generalist. Not only

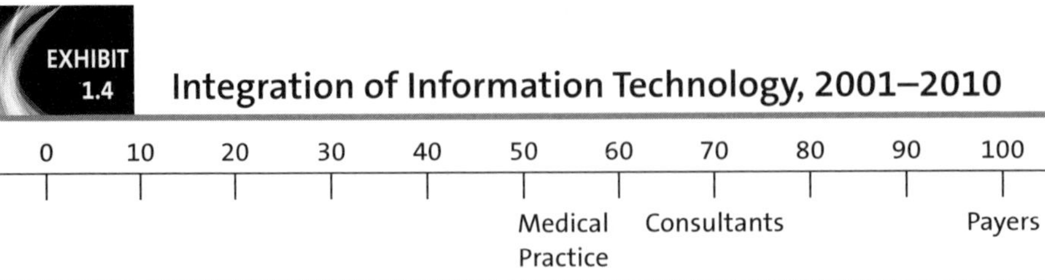

does it put the ICA in a position to negotiate based upon size distribution, it also benefits them from the perspective of having a knowledge base of information. The latter allows them to more effectively and efficiently diagnose and treat the problems found in the most complex of medical practice issues.

As you work within the new millennium, you will continue to see a dramatic shift in the overall picture of how the successful medical practice and, consequently, the healthcare consultant will work (see Exhibit 1.4). IT and business integration will no longer be an option for those on the cutting edge. It will be a necessity for everyone because of total integration on the payer side. From this, there is a great paradox that follows. The traditionalist healthcare provider who leaves practice because of an inability or unwillingness to go along with the program has a slim chance of reentering healthcare from a horizontal perspective. In other words, the traditionalist's chances of staying in healthcare on the nonclinical side, such as administration, management, or consulting, are weak. This is mainly because of the very reason that the provider left in the first place. Traditionalism has no place in a highly dynamic industry. The second reason is that most providers, because of the sheltering they may have experienced in the past, have been prohibited from having the "big picture" view. Although it may seem offensive to some, my personal opinion is this: either embrace change and learn to rapidly adapt or learn to say, "would you like fries with that." From the perspective of the training and education required to become a physician, it is an all-or-none proposition.

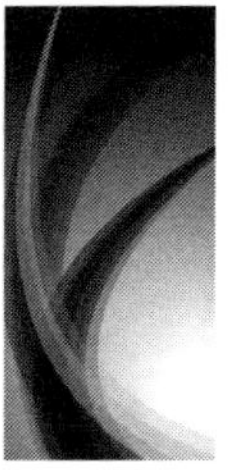

CHAPTER 2

The Essentials of the Resource-Based Relative Value Scale

In order to compete effectively within the marketplace, it is essential that the practice understand the foundational components of the resource-based relative value scale. Although not everyone agrees on the methodological approach to the scale's development and maintenance, it has become the standard in the industry for application of specific financial, analytical, and statistical studies.

A relative value scale is a database model that is used to measure the value of a service, procedure, or product relative to the value of another service, procedure, or product.

WHAT IS A RELATIVE VALUE SCALE?

Most simply put, a relative value scale, in any setting, is a quantifiable model used to assign a specific fee or other value to a service, procedure, or product based upon the value of another service, procedure, or product. In the automobile industry, for example, an estimate that is given to a customer for repair of his or her vehicle is usually based upon what is called a "flat rate" book, or the Chilton's Manual. This book lists the average expected hours required to perform a given repair for a specific vehicle type, make, model, and year. This estimate of hours is then multiplied by the hourly rate to obtain the fee for the estimated repair.

When applying the relative value scale to the healthcare industry, there are also two components used to decide the fee for a particular procedure. The first is known as a relative value unit, or RVU. As the name describes, this is a unit of measurement that stipulates the value for a specific procedure or service relative to other procedures or services. The RVU is used to determine complexity, consumption of resources, and, with respect to billing and reimbursement, the fee for that procedure or service.

In healthcare, the relative value unit measures both the relative complexity of the procedure and the consumption of resources. Some have come to believe that the relative value unit measures productivity, but this is not the case.

The conversion factor is the value that is used to "convert" the relative value unit into a fee. The federal government sets the conversion factor for Medicare each year, but the conversion factor for each procedure will vary for most practices.

The higher the RVU value, the more time and effort expended, the higher the cost and, for the most part, the greater the complexity and consumption of resources, and, finally, the higher the fee. For example, an office visit for an established patient may only be calculated at 1 RVU, and open-heart surgery may be calculated at 100 RVUs. In this case, the RVU for the heart surgery reflects that the procedure consumes 100 times the resources and has a fee that is 100 times greater than the office visit.

The next component is called the conversion factor (CF). The CF is a dollar value that is used to "convert" the RVU value into a fee. For example, for Medicare, the CF for 2012 was 34.0376.* This means that each RVU under the resource-based relative value scale (RBRVS) system was equivalent to approximately $34.04. So, for an office visit for an established patient that is equal to 1 RVU, the fee would be established at $34.04 (without adjustment for geographic locality). For the open-heart surgical procedure assigned 100 RVUs, the fee would be established at $3,4037.60. Therefore, to calculate a fee for any given procedure, multiply the CF by the RVU. Inversely, if the fee and the RVU are known, you could obtain the CF by dividing the fee by the RVU.

WHAT IS THE RESOURCE-BASED RELATIVE VALUE SCALE?

A resource-based relative value scale is specific in that it uses the consumption of resources as a basis for its methodology. Before 1998, the practice expense component of the resource-based relative value scale was based on cost. As of 2002, it is only based on resources.

The RBRVS is a relative value scale that is based upon the consumption of resources and not a historical or empirical measurement of value. The RBRVS is broken into three distinct components, called RVUs, or relative value units, each measuring a different component of the procedure or service being performed or provided for or on behalf of the patient. The three components are work RVU, practice expense RVU, and malpractice RVU. The total RVU is calculated as the sum of these individual components.

The RBRVS was developed by the Cambridge Health Economics Group for use by the Centers for Medicare & Medicaid Services (CMS), formerly the Health Care Financing Administration (HCFA), the government agency that oversees the Medicare program. The primary use for the RBRVS is in determining reimbursement rates for physicians under the Medicare payment system, or the Physician Fee Schedule Database.

* This edition of *RVUs: Applications for Medical Practice Success* was written in 2012 and examples throughout the book are based on 2012 values. Also, values within examples and exhibits have been rounded for ease of use.

HISTORY OF THE RESOURCE-BASED RELATIVE VALUE SCALE

Prior to development of the RBRVS, the universally accepted method of reimbursement was based upon usual, customary, and reasonable (UCR) charges (also known as customary, prevailing, and reasonable charges). Until the advent of the RBRVS, even the existing relative value scales were based upon physicians' charges, which simply perpetuated the market's price distortions. Because of the variation in charges and payments due, in large part, to the geographic variability and the fiscal constraints imposed by Medicare in the mid-1970s and early 1980s, some physicians' dissatisfaction with the UCR system increased. For others, such as surgeons, the UCR system was quite satisfactory because surgeries were high revenue producers and quite profitable in many cases.

Requests to change and improve the system of reimbursement began with physicians, the American Medical Association (AMA), insurance companies, and the government; however, this change began predominantly with primary care organizations that were faced with an increasing shortfall in revenues under UCR. It was clear that with UCR, there was little equivalence between evaluation and management (E/M) services and surgical services.

In 1985, HCFA contracted with the Harvard University School of Public Health to develop objective measures of physician work. Outcomes would provide a more acceptable and perhaps more competitive payment system for physicians across all specialties providing care to Medicare beneficiaries. Over the next three years, a multidisciplinary research team, headed by Dr. William C. Hsiao, conducted a national study that resulted in the development of the methodology behind the RBRVS. Although the methodology included calculating the effort of providing each procedure in terms of physician work, practice expense, and professional liability, the primary objective of the Harvard study was to measure physician work rather than all three components.

In this study, a cross section of physicians determined the relative amount of work, time, and effort that encompassed various procedures they performed. Relative to *what* was the original challenge. Current Procedural Terminology (CPT; CPT codes are a copyright of the American Medical Association) code 99213, which is the code for an established patient office visit with face-to-face time with a physician lasting approximately 15 minutes, was the anchor code from which the entire RBRVS was developed. At the genesis of the RBRVS, the total number of RVUs assigned to CPT 99213 was 1.0. It has, however, changed over the years. For 2012, the unadjusted total non-facility RVU for 99213 was 2.07, and the work RVU hovered near the 1.0 mark, at 0.97. The physicians' task was to determine what value should be assigned to other codes relative to 99213 and its value of 1.0. Thus began the process of the RBRVS development.

As part of the study, technical consulting groups (TCGs) comprising more than 200 physicians were organized into 33 specialty-specific consulting groups to provide guidance on the study structure and to define physician work. Vignettes were created to specifically describe the clinical content of each service so that uniform definitions could be written and clearly understood by all physicians nationwide. The TCGs defined physicians' total work as encompassing both time and intensity. Intensity included mental effort, clinical judgment, technical skill, physical effort, and iatrogenic stress related to risk. Iatrogenic risk is defined as an inadvertent adverse effect or complication as a result of medical treatment. Total work was divided into three time periods: pre-service, intra-service, and post-service. In an attempt to provide a readily defensible method of valuing "work effort," magnitude estimation, which is a way of measuring subjective perceptions and judgments, was used to measure physicians' subjective perceptions of procedure time and complexity when rating services. The use of magnitude estimation proved to be reliable and produced valid results in previous studies.

A resource-based relative value scale analysis by itself does not have much value. It is when the results are applied to other models that the value of this type of analysis shines through.

One year after the study results were submitted to HCFA for use in the Medicare payment system, President George H. W. Bush signed the Omnibus Budget Reconciliation Act of 1989 into law, which switched Medicare to an RBRVS payment system effective Jan. 1, 1992. Voilà! The Medicare Physicians' Fee Schedule (MPFS) was born. Updated between once and a dozen times a year since 1992, the RBRVS, upon which the MPFS is based, has evolved into an industry standard for physician practice metrics and assessments.

Section 1848, Payment for Physician Services, of the Social Security Act addresses Medicare payments for services rendered by physicians. It mandates that payments be made based upon national, uniform RVUs and that a sustainable growth rate be maintained for the rates of increase in Medicare payments.

Today, the annual updates recommended to CMS for the work component of the RBRVS RVUs come primarily from the Relative Value Scale

Update Committee (RUC), a 29-member expert panel formed by the AMA. The RUC represents the entire medical profession with 23 of its 29 membership seats appointed by major national medical specialty societies. Three of those specialties rotate membership every two years. Two seats are reserved for internal medicine subspecialties, and one seat is open to any other medical specialty. The remaining six seats are reserved for the RUC chair, the Practice Expense Review Committee chair, the Health Care Professionals Advisory Committee co-chair, and representatives from the AMA, the American Osteopathic Association, and the CPT Editorial Panel. Additional information on the RUC, RVUs, and the history of the RBRVS can be found on the AMA Web site (www.ama-assn.org).

Until 2002, not all three RVU components were resource based. In the beginning, only the work component was resource based. So even though the scale has always been called the "resource-based relative value scale," the term was a bit of a misnomer. Until the late 1990s, HCFA computed the practice expense and the professional liability components using a formula that included average Medicare-approved charges. In 2000, the last of the three components, the malpractice component, was converted from actual claims-paid data values to resource-based values. Each RVU component is scheduled for comprehensive five-year reviews, so changes over time are inevitable. In 2007, the practice expense component had its five-year review, resulting in a complete change in methodology.

All three RVU components became fully resource based in 2002.

The Medicare reimbursement for the practice expense component was originally calculated by multiplying a percentage of gross revenues that a specialty practice spent on overhead (practice expenses) by the historical payment for a procedure or service. Resource-based practice expense values were phased in over a four-year period, which was completed in 2002. The transitional methodology, which was designed to smooth the implementation process, was organized as follows:

- Year 1: 75 percent of the original method plus 25 percent of the new method
- Year 2: 50 percent of the original method plus 50 percent of the new method
- Year 3: 25 percent of the original method plus 75 percent of the new method
- Year 4: 100 percent is the new method.

In 2007, just as healthcare administrators had become accustomed to how their Medicare payments were calculated, CMS again revised the methodology behind the practice expense values and began phasing it in over another four-year period, which ended in 2010, with a similar transitional methodology. Why? CMS wanted to provide a more transparent methodology than the previous one in order to allow medical practices to "predict the effects of proposals to improve accuracy of practice expense payments." This methodology comprised a bottom-up approach for direct costs and supplementary survey data for indirect costs. The nonphysician work pool previously included in the overhead RVU has been eliminated. The nonphysician work pool was a special method used to calculate practice expense RVUs for services associated with nonphysician work.

Then, just when you thought it was over, another major change occurred effective 2010. This change, which affects the practice expense RVU, necessitated another four-year transition. Overall, the practice expense component represents, on average, close to 44 percent of the total RVUs for each service. In this third four-year transition, which began in 2010, CMS engaged in additional practice expense revisions using the results of the Physician Practice Information Survey, sponsored by AMA and other healthcare organizations, and an assumption that diagnostic imaging equipment is in use closer to 90 percent of the time that the office is open rather than 50 percent of the time. The transitional methodology is, once again, the same blended model you experienced in the past two; it had a proposed full implementation date of Jan. 1, 2013.

It is clear that this database is a moving target in reference to time. As such, for the purposes of this book, I use the fully implemented, nongeographically adjusted RVU values, which was expected to be effective in 2013.

When using RBRVS to conduct studies and analyses within your own practice, I recommend that you use the transitioned RVUs because these are the values that would be effective for that particular (current) time period. You can ignore the fully implemented practice expense values because they are not used in calculations and only show what the RVUs will be in 2013 when the four-year transition is complete. These fully implemented values are likely to change again. So, in the meantime, stick with the transitioned values! The database will look something like Exhibit 2.1.

CMS's RBRVS is composed of Health Care Financing Administration Current Procedural Coding System (HCPCS) codes, which are broken into three levels;

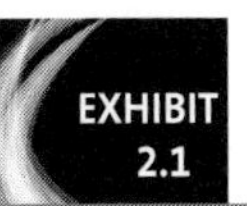
EXHIBIT 2.1

Sample of RBRVS Database Downloaded from CMS

HCPCS MOD	NOT USED FOR MEDICARE WORK PAYMENT RVU	TRANSITIONED NON-FAC PE RVU	FULLY IMPLEMENTED NON-FAC PE RVU	TRANSITIONED FACILITY PE RVU	FULLY IMPLEMENTED FACILITY PE RVU	MP RVU	TRANSITIONED NON-FACILITY TOTAL	FULLY IMPLEMENTED NON-FACILITY TOTAL	TRANSITIONED FACILITY TOTAL	FULLY IMPLEMENTED FACILITY TOTAL
48540	21.94	11.55	12.06	11.55	12.06	4.67	38.16	38.67	38.16	38.67
48545	22.23	12.16	12.75	12.16	12.75	4.75	39.14	39.73	39.14	39.73
48547	30.38	15.36	16.05	15.36	16.05	6.46	52.20	52.89	52.20	52.89
48548	28.09	14.46	14.99	14.46	14.99	5.97	48.52	49.05	48.52	49.05
48550	0.00	0.00	0.00	0.00	0.00	0.00	0.00	0.00	0.00	0.00
48551	0.00	0.00	0.00	0.00	0.00	0.00	0.00	0.00	0.00	0.00
48552	4.30	1.70	1.74	1.70	1.74	0.90	6.90	6.94	6.90	6.94
48554	37.80	28.90	30.09	28.90	30.09	7.89	74.59	75.78	74.59	75.78
48556	19.47	13.48	14.08	13.48	14.08	4.15	37.10	37.70	37.10	37.70
48999	0.00	0.00	0.00	0.00	0.00	0.00	0.00	0.00	0.00	0.00
49000	12.54	7.40	7.63	7.40	7.63	2.57	22.51	22.74	22.51	22.74
49002	17.63	9.14	9.59	9.14	9.59	3.66	30.43	30.88	30.43	30.88
49010	16.06	8.33	8.47	8.33	8.47	3.20	27.59	27.73	27.59	27.73
49020	26.67	14.30	14.81	14.30	14.81	5.42	46.90	46.90	46.39	46.90

- Level I is made up of the CPT codes, brief descriptions, and the RVUs associated with each code.
- Level II codes are maintained by CMS for reporting products, supplies, and services not included in the CPT codes, such as ambulance services and durable medical equipment, prosthetics, orthotics, and supplies, when used outside a physician's office. Unlike CPT codes, which are either all numeric (or at least begin with a number), HCPCS level II codes are alphanumeric, with the first position of each code an alpha between A and W.
- Level III codes are considered specific to a local carrier. These codes are also alphanumeric and begin with an X, Y, or Z. Level III codes are not included in the national policy and therefore are not assigned RVU values.

The RBRVS is not copyrighted because its source is a federal government agency and it is therefore considered public domain. As previously mentioned, the AMA holds the copyright to the CPT codes. This has been a source of some confusion in the past because people often think of the RBRVS and RVUs as being synonymous, while in reality the RVUs constitute only one part of the entire RBRVS.

Finally, lest you think that the RBRVS is the pinnacle of health services measurement, it should be pointed out that the current RBRVS has limitations. Although inputs are carefully measured, the RBRVS does not consider or include adjustments for healthcare outcomes (i.e., output), severity, quality of care, or demand for services. RVUs do not account for practice efficiencies or inefficiencies. In addition, not all codes (e.g., laboratory and HCPCS) have RVUs assigned. This makes it more difficult to place a standardized value on those procedures and/or services. As Salvador Dali said, "Have no fear of perfection; you'll never reach it." So it is true with RVUs, which continue to evolve with health services.

However, because the RBRVS is a relational model, when used within the universe of a closed entity, such as a practice or system, it is incredibly effective at measuring costs, resource expenditures, fees, and productivity. Those codes that do not have RVU values assigned, such as some lab procedures and many of the J codes (drugs), lack RVUs for a reason. By themselves, they do not consume a resource related to anything other than supply cost. Drugs, for example, don't do anything to warrant a value. The administration of the drug, however, does. And when conducting RBRVS-based cost analyses, you will see that the separation of non-RVU procedures provides an overall more accurate outcome.

USE OF THE RESOURCE-BASED RELATIVE VALUE SCALE

With the exception of cursory reviews for relationships of fees to the Medicare fee schedule (MFS) amount, a RBRVS analysis alone provides little useful information for the typical medical practice. Because each medical practice is distinct in its financial and operational structure, the RBRVS is not a very good model for benchmarking across disparate medical practices. Within a closed universe, however, such as within a practice entity, the RBRVS is very effective for benchmarking specific markers within the practice and for use in developing other valuable financial, operational, statistical, and utilization models. These models include the following:

- Development of fees for new and existing practices
- Procedural and global cost accounting
- Resource allocation
- Physician productivity and compensation issues
- General practice productivity studies

- Break-even and profit/loss analysis
- Managed care contract analysis
- Per member per month capitation cost analysis
- Global pricing
- Compliance risk

The relative value unit is made up of three distinct components as is the geographical adjustment factor. These three components, factored together, will determine the total adjusted relative value unit for a procedure.

UNDERSTANDING THE RESOURCE-BASED RELATIVE VALUE SCALE MODEL

The RBRVS incorporates three major component concepts that are used to perform its calculations. The first is referred to as a *relative value unit*, or RVU. The total RVU is composed of three subcomponents, which will be discussed later in this chapter. The RVU is assigned a value for the provision of each medical service or procedure. The next component concept is the *geographic adjustment factor*, or GAF. Like the RVU, the GAF is composed of three subcomponents, called geographic practice cost indices (GPCI), each of which corresponds to the RVU subcomponents. The GPCIs are mathematically applied to factor in cost differences in operating medical practices in different parts of the country. The final component is the *conversion factor*, or CF. The CF measures the per-unit dollar value for each RVU, converting it from a relative value into a fee or an actual charge. The CF is valuable in other areas of the medical practice and will be discussed in detail later in this text.

Relative Value Components

RVUs are nonmonetary, relative units of measure that report the relative differences in resources consumed when providing various procedures and services. Many people see RBRVS as an objective, standardized method for analyzing resources involved in the provision of services or procedures. This, however, is not necessarily true. Within the three components of the RBRVS, the practice expense RVU is influenced by subjective political and financial reasons, and there is a great deal of disagreement as to whether an RVU methodology really provides a method for equitable payment for medical services rendered to patients. RVUs assign *relative* values, or weights, to medical procedures primarily for the purpose of establishing a budget-neutral system of payment under the Medicare program. Period! The fact that RVUs are used for other purposes, such as cost modeling, performance, and compensation, is secondary. And the fact that so many

The three distinct components that make up the total relative value unit are:

- *Work*
- *Practice expense*
- *Malpractice*

payers depend on RVUs to develop and maintain fee schedules is just plain wrong. RVUs can also be used to assist practices in both internal benchmarking within departments and external benchmarking against similar groups and external metrics.

Perhaps of critical importance is to remember that the RVU, in the absence of a conversion factor (discussed later), has no financial value whatsoever. RVUs do not measure value. RVUs do not measure productivity. RVUs do not measure waste. RVUs measure—and only measure—the degree to which all resources are consumed.

Work Relative Value Unit Component

The first RVU component, in order of appearance, is the *work* component (RVU_{WK}). Work RVUs are designed to measure the time and effort expended by the provider in the delivery of the service or procedure. The time category is composed of three subcategories. Pre-service time accounts for things such as prep time, waiting time, pre-surgical example, etc. Intra-service time reports the interaction between the patient and the provider. Face-to-face time describes this interaction in nonsurgical situations, such as with E/M visits. Skin-to-skin time describes this interaction in surgical situations, during which the provider is actively engaged in the procedure itself. Post-service time describes the time during which the provider (or his/her representative) provides follow-up care to the patient. Normally, the duration of post-service time is part of the CMS guidelines based on the specific procedure being performed. Each of these refers to a separate and distinct part of the total time spent for that procedure.

The second subcategory (intensity) refers to the mental effort and judgment, technical skill, physical effort, and iatrogenic risk involved in delivering the service. When aggregated, the work RVU is designed to measure the average total work by a physician of average efficiency and average skill and training as well as measure the consumption of the provider's resources. The Harvard/RUC Time Study has a major influence on the development of the value for this subcomponent. Later, I discuss how this study can also be used in physician productivity applications to develop full-time equivalent definitions and measure assessed time.

Practice Expense Relative Value Unit Component

One method of differentiating among the different ways of calculating the practice component RVUs is to classify an approach as either "top down" or "bottom up." A top-down approach starts by estimating a practice expense pool for a set of physician services and then allocating that pool to each individual procedure or service at the code level. This is in contrast to a bottom-up approach where practice expenses are first developed, code by code, for a set of reference services. Next, practice expenses for non-referenced services are imputed. Finally, practice expenses are totaled across codes and then calibrated to correspond to an overall budget target (the practice expense pool).

CMS adopted a top-down approach using two data sources to establish its practice expense pool: the AMA's Socioeconomic Monitoring System (SMS) and the Clinical Practice Expert Panel (CPEP). CMS used data derived from the 1995 through 1997 SMS surveys to create the direct and indirect physician specialty-specific practice expense pools. The CPEP data were used to allocate the direct expense pools across the services paid under the Medicare physician fee schedule, while the indirect pools were allocated to individual codes using the work RVUs and the direct expense information. Additional information needed to implement the practice expense methodology is obtained from the following four sources: AMA's specialty society RUC, surveys done by Harvard for the initial establishment of the work RVUs, work RVUs, and Medicare physician claims database. This section includes a brief review of how each component is used to construct resource-based practice expense RVUs, and some of the issues considered in this book are introduced.

There are two major steps required to attain these values. The first is the process of creating the practice expense pools and the second involves the process of actually calculating total physician hours. Total hours per procedure by specialty were calculated as the product of the time it takes to perform a procedure, obtained from the RUC data, and the frequency of that procedure, obtained from the Medicare claims data. These hours were then aggregated across procedures for each specialty. The practice expense pools are created by taking the total practice expenses in the pool and dividing by the total reported physician hours. This equals the average practice expense per hour. Practice expenses per hour were then averaged across all responding physician owners within each specialty.

The second stage of the practice expense methodology allocates expense pools across the procedure codes. HCFA used different allocation approaches for direct and indirect costs. The direct cost pools include practice expenses for clinical labor, medical supplies, and medical equipment. Direct costs were allocated using procedure-level CPEP cost data on clinical labor, medical supplies, and medical equipment. The indirect cost pools include practice expenses for administrative labor, office supplies, and other expenses. Indirect costs were allocated across the procedure codes using a combination of the code-level direct practice expenses and physician work RVUs.

Malpractice Expense Relative Value Unit Component

The third and final component is known as the *malpractice expense* component of the relative value unit (RVU_{MP}). This subcomponent is intended to measure the cost of malpractice insurance based upon specialty; however, it does not do this. Therefore, the name for this component is somewhat misleading. Rather, it is used to measure the relative risk to the provider and the relative cost for training a physician as a result of their specific specialty. Therefore, procedures that would be performed primarily by a physician with a specific specialty would reflect these factors in the RVU_{MP} component. In addition, it also represents the income forgone when physicians pursue additional years of specialty training rather than entering practice right away, which is why surgical services have a higher malpractice RVU than an office visit.

When all three components are added together for any given procedure, the total RVU is determined. As you will learn in the next few paragraphs, however, this total represents a national average for that total RVU because it has not yet been adjusted for geographic location.

Just like the relative value unit, the geographic adjustment factor *is broken down into the same three components: work, practice, and malpractice. These components determine the difference in these three areas based upon geographical location.*

► Geographic Adjustment Factor Components

For the purpose of the RBRVS as it was applied to Medicare, a geographical component called the geographic adjustment factor was developed to adjust the financial value of each component of the procedure by specific geographic factors. The GAF is broken into three subcomponents known as geographic practice cost indices, or the GPCIs. The GPCIs are used to determine the GAF for each Medicare location. For 2012, there were 90 of these localities in which all but 16 states are statewide localities, meaning every physician in the state receives the same Medicare payment amount. The remaining states have more than one locality. The concept is that localities that, for the most part, consist of a state's major urban areas receive higher reimbursement rates than paid in the rest of the state. This is not, however, the case. In fact, the GAF is a poorly designed method that, if anything, aggregates resource data rather than segregates resource data, resulting in a penalty to higher-cost areas and bonuses to lower-cost areas. For example, the state of Ohio has only one GAF. It's pretty obvious to both residents and nonresidents of Ohio that there are both major and minor financial divisions within the state, and one common factor does nothing to enhance the demarcation of those geographic definitions. Florida, on the other hand, has three GAF locations: Fort Lauderdale, Miami, and rest of Florida, which includes metropolitan areas such as Tampa-Clearwater-St. Petersburg, Jacksonville, Gainesville, and Orlando, while at the same time including more rural areas such as Chiefland, Palatka, and Lake City. It should be obvious to even the casual observer that the GAF model is broken and badly in need of a more thoughtful and analytical approach.

The GAF, like the RVU, is broken down into three distinct subcomponents. They correspond to the RVU subcomponents in name and purpose and are described in the following paragraphs.

Work Component of the Geographic Adjustment Factor

The work component of the GAF (GAF_{WK}) is used to adjust for the opportunity cost of physician time and effort. Strictly speaking, the opportunity costs of physician time and effort would involve the income a physician could earn if he or she had entered an alternative learned profession. In fact, the GPCI adjustment for physician time and effort involves estimates for each locality (relative to the national average) of the median hourly earnings of professionals who have had at least five years of college.

Practice Expense Component of the Geographic Adjustment Factor

The GAF_{PE} measures the supposed actual difference between measurable expense categories based upon the specific geographic location listed in the GPCI table. These would include such factors as the cost for electricity and other utilities, hourly wages for specific healthcare-related Standard Industrial Classification (SIC) categories, lease expense for professional office space, and similar expenses.

Malpractice Expense Component of the Geographic Adjustment Factor

The GAF_{MP} is designed to measure the actual cost of malpractice and professional liability insurance for that specific location and/or area.

Unfortunately, this factor is updated every two years even though, in many locations, the cost of malpractice may rise quarterly. This subcomponent does not fairly or adequately represent the malpractice expense that many physicians are facing today and should, in my opinion, be renamed.

CALCULATING THE ADJUSTED RELATIVE VALUE UNIT

To get the total geographically adjusted relative value unit, factor each relative value unit component by each **geographic adjustment factor** *component and then add them together.*

The total RVU value can be calculated in two ways. First, it can be determined by adding the three components together without factoring in the GAF, resulting in a geographically neutral value. Second, it can be calculated by first factoring in the GAF, resulting in what is called a geographically adjusted RVU. The second method is used exclusively to determine the MFS amount. In this case, instead of factoring the total RVU with the total GAF, each subcomponent is factored first and then the geographically adjusted RVU is obtained by getting the sum of those products.

To calculate the adjusted total RVU amount for an existing procedure, first factor in each GAF with the corresponding RVU, as follows:

$$\text{Geographically Adjusted Total RVU} = [(\text{Work RVU} * \text{Work GPCI}) + (\text{Practice Expense RVU} * \text{Practice Expense GPCI}) + (\text{Malpractice RVU} * \text{Malpractice GPCI})]$$

Then take the sum of the products to get the total. Here is an example using procedure code 99213 for the region "rest of Florida":

$$[(RVU_W * GPCI_W) + (RVU_{PE} * GPCI_{PE}) + (RVU_{MP} * GPCI_{MP})] =$$
$$(.097 * 1.00) + (1.03 * 0.968) + (0.07 * 0.553) =$$
$$0.097 + 0.997 + 0.0387 =$$

The sum of the products is 1.133 total geographically adjusted RVUs.

To obtain the Medicare fee schedule amount, multiply the geographically adjusted total relative value unit times the Medicare conversion factor for the current year.

CALCULATING THE MEDICARE FEE SCHEDULE AMOUNT

The MFS amount is the amount that the CMS will allow in calculating reimbursement for the medical provider. There are two distinct reimbursement methodologies, depending upon whether the physician is designated as a participating or nonparticipating provider. The latter is reimbursed on what is known as the limiting charge, indicating that the amount that is actually billed to Medicare is limited by a specific mathematical formula. A participating physician may bill Medicare any amount, making it easier to maintain a single fee schedule for the practice. A caveat here is that a medical provider should bill Medicare substantially more than they bill private payers.

The Medicare limiting charge is set by law at 115 percent of the MFS amount for the service furnished by the nonparticipating physician. However, the law sets the amount reimbursed to the provider by Medicare for nonparticipating physicians at 95 percent of the payment amount for participating physicians (i.e., the fee schedule amount). Multiplying 95 percent of the 80 percent paid to participating providers is equivalent to multiplying the allowed amount by a factor of .76 (or 76 percent). Therefore, to calculate the Medicare reimbursement for a non-par physician service for a locality, multiply the fee schedule amount by a factor of .76. The provider may then balance-bill the patient the difference between the 76 percent of the allowed amount and the 115 percent that represents the limiting charge. Sound confusing? It is meant to be. There are other penalties for being a nonparticipating physician, and CMS's goal, through a series of incentives and disincentives, is to have all medical providers participate in the Medicare program. (As of 2010, about 87 percent of all physicians had signed up for participation status.)

To obtain the MFS amount, multiply the total geographically adjusted RVU by the Medicare CF for that given year, as follows:

$$\text{MFS} = \text{RVU}_{\text{TOT}} * \text{Medicare CF}$$

Using the example above and the current CF of 34.0376, the calculation would look like this:

$$\text{MFS} = 1.133 * 34.0376 = \$38.56$$

Many practices have asked why they should bother to calculate the MFS for their practice because it is available from the carrier and published and distributed each year. The answer is simple: often what is published and reimbursed by the carriers is wrong. On many occasions, a carrier is allowed a different amount (always less) than the correct amount. By calculating your own MFS allowable and comparing that number to the number your carrier publishes, you can ensure that you are getting paid what you are entitled to under the Medicare program.

FACILITY VS. NON-FACILITY PROCEDURES

Procedures performed within the actual practice location are subject to reimbursement as a non-facility charge. Procedures performed at a location other than the medical office are considered facility charges and are reimbursed for a smaller amount. The only difference in the relative value unit calculations is the practice expense component.

In 1998, CMS released two practice expense components. One was for calculating the fee when a procedure was performed in the physician's office and the other was used to calculate the fee if the procedure was performed anywhere except the physician's office or a location designated as the physician's office. Not all procedure codes were represented by this site-of-service (SOS) differential. In fact, only about 650 codes had differences in the value for the practice expense component.

Under the resource-based system, this policy is no longer applicable because, where appropriate, CMS has developed practice expense RVUs specific to the facility and non-facility settings. In this case, it is only the practice expense RVU subcomponent that is affected. In those situations where the definition applies, the practice expense subcomponent will generally be less for facility-based charges and therefore more for non-facility–based charges.

Generally, under the resource-based system, the facility practice expense RVUs will be used for services performed in inpatient or outpatient hospital settings, emergency rooms, skilled nursing facilities, or ambulatory surgical centers (ASCs). The non-facility practice expense RVUs generally will be used for services furnished in a physician's office, patient's home, or a residential living facility.

Note that a procedure performed in an ASC that is not on the ASC list is reimbursed on the basis of the non-facility practice expense RVUs. Outpatient rehabilitation services usually will be reimbursed based on the non-facility practice expense RVUs.

Non-facility: A non-facility designation is assigned to a procedure or service that is delivered within the medical practice or an extension thereof. The location is determined on the CMS-1500 billing form in box 24. The assumption is that if the physician delivers the service within the office or another location where she or he has a fair market value financial burden, she or he is entitled to a higher reimbursement amount for consumption of resources such as electricity, staff, and supplies.

Facility: Unlike its similarly named counterpart, this refers to a factoring used to determine a provider charge under the Medicare outpatient (Part B) payment system, *not* the amount charged by a facility such as a hospital or ASC. This factor is used whenever the provider delivers the procedure or service in a setting other than the physician's office or associated extension thereof. This may include facilities such as nursing homes, hospitals, and ASCs. The assumption is that the provider is not consuming his or her own office resources, so is not entitled to as much reimbursement.

CMS did not develop non-facility practice expense RVUs for some services that, either by definition or in practice, are never (or rarely) performed in a non-facility setting. For example, by definition, the initial hospital care codes (99221–99223) are provided only in the hospital inpatient setting. Also, many major surgical procedures with a 90-day global period are almost always performed in the hospital inpatient setting. An "NA" identifies these facility-only codes in the NA Indicator field of the final physician fee schedule addendum B, published in the *Federal Register*. Effective CY 2004, CMS has assigned the facility value to the non-facility RVU for procedures previously assigned the NA designation. The same is true for assignment of facility RVU values for non-facility procedures previously assigned the NA designation.

SAMPLE GEOGRAPHIC ADJUSTMENT FACTORS AND RELATIVE VALUE UNIT VALUES

Pick a code from addendum B of the Federal Register *and the geographic adjustment factor from addendum D and try this for yourself.*

Let's calculate the total adjusted RVU and RBRVS fee amount for procedure code 99203 for the Miami designated region.

The GAF for this area is:

Work component 1.000

Practice expense component 1.054

Malpractice component 2.815

For procedure code 99203, the RVU components are as follows:

Work component 1.42

Non-facility practice expense component 1.53

Facility practice expense component 0.64

Malpractice component 0.14

Note that for the GPCI values, a number greater than 1 represents the ratio by which the factored expenses are greater than that of the national

In the non-facility calculation, you use the non-facility practice expense component. Note that facility and non-facility definitions do not have an effect on the geographic adjustment factor components.

average. For example, the malpractice component above, at 2.815, indicates that the cost of risk for physicians in Miami is approximately 2.8 times higher than the national average for that same metric.

SAMPLE NON-FACILITY RELATIVE VALUE UNIT CALCULATION

Using the above data set, calculate the non-facility total adjusted RVU as follows:

$$(RVU_{WK} * GAF_{WK}) + (\text{non-facility } RVU_{PE} * GAF_{PE}) + (RVU_{MP} * GAF_{MP}) = RVU_{TOT}$$

$$(1.42 * 1.000) + (1.53 * 1.054) + (0.14 * 2.815)$$

$$1.42 + 1.61 + 0.39$$

This equals the geographically adjusted non-facility total RVU of 3.42.

To obtain the MFS allowable amount, multiply the RVU_{TOT} times the current year Medicare CF as follows:

$$3.42 * \$34.0376 = \$116.41$$

In calculating the facility relative value unit, use the facility practice expense component of the relative value unit. Note that the difference between the facility and non-facility fee amounts equals $28.81.

SAMPLE FACILITY RELATIVE VALUE UNIT CALCULATION

Using the above data set, calculate for the facility total adjusted RVU as follows:

$$(RVU_{WK} * GAF_{WK}) + (\text{Facility } RVU_{PE} * GAF_{PE}) + (RVU_{MP} * GAF_{MP}) = RVU_{TOT}$$

$$(1.42 * 1.000) + (0.64 * 1.054) + (0.14 * 2.815)$$

$$1.42 + 0.67 + 0.39$$

This equals the geographically adjusted non-facility total RVU of 2.48.

To obtain the approximate Medicare fee amount, multiply the RVU_{TOT} times the CF as follows:

$$2.48 * \$34.0376 = \$84.41$$

Note again that the only difference between the facility and non-facility calculation is the value of the practice expense RVU.

BUILDING THE RESOURCE-BASED RELATIVE VALUE SCALE TABLE

To build an RBRVS, first develop a spreadsheet that contains all of the RVU values for each procedure code you wish to analyze (Exhibit 2.2).

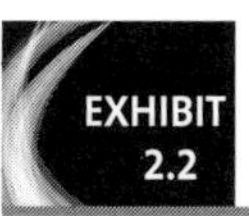

EXHIBIT 2.2 Initial Build for RBRVS Spreadsheet

HCPCS Code	Work RVU	Non-Facility Practice Expense RVU	Facility Practice Expense RVU	Malpractice RVU
10040	1.18	0.583	0.270	0.020
10060	1.17	0.650	0.325	0.030
10061	2.40	0.965	0.530	0.050
10080	1.17	0.838	0.353	0.040
10081	2.45	1.480	0.768	0.130
10120	1.22	0.765	0.338	0.040
10121	2.69	1.428	0.778	0.090
10140	1.53	0.695	0.388	0.040
10160	1.20	0.640	0.320	0.040
10180	2.25	1.153	1.140	0.140

There are two types of modifiers: those that affect reimbursement and those that don't. It is important to factor the relative value unit using the same reimbursement relationship that exists between the modified procedure and its nonmodified global counterpart.

► Adjust Totals for Geographic Adjustment Factor Values

Next, using the following GPCI values and selected practice expense components, adjust the total RVU amounts (Exhibit 2.3).

Work = 0.975 Practice Expense = 0.946 Malpractice = 1.268

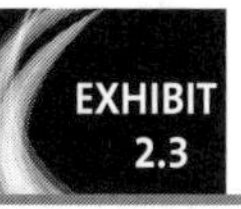

EXHIBIT 2.3 Table of GPCI-Adjusted RVU Values

HCPCS Code	Work RVU	Non-Facility Practice Expense RVU	Facility Practice Expense RVU	Malpractice RVU	Total Non-Facility RVU	Total Facility RVU	Adjusted Non-Facility RVU	Adjusted Facility RVU
10040	1.18	0.583	0.270	0.020	1.783	1.470	1.727	1.431
10060	1.17	0.650	0.325	0.030	1.850	1.525	1.794	1.486
10061	2.40	0.965	0.530	0.050	3.415	2.980	3.316	2.905
10080	1.17	0.838	0.353	0.040	2.048	1.563	1.984	1.525
10081	2.45	1.480	0.768	0.130	4.060	3.348	3.954	3.280
10120	1.22	0.765	0.338	0.040	2.025	1.598	1.964	1.559
10121	2.69	1.428	0.778	0.090	4.208	3.558	4.087	3.472
10140	1.53	0.695	0.388	0.040	2.265	1.958	2.200	1.909
10160	1.20	0.640	0.320	0.040	1.880	1.560	1.826	1.523
10180	2.25	1.153	1.140	0.140	3.543	3.530	3.462	3.450

Calculate the Medicare Fee Schedule Amount

Finally, using the current CF, multiply the selected adjusted practice expense components to get the MFS amounts (Exhibit 2.4).

Medicare conversion factor = $34.0376

Modifier-Factored Relative Value Units

Most medical practices regularly use one or more modifiers. A modifier is a two-character alphanumeric designation that identifies a modification or change to the global procedure code. The use of the modifier does not change the description of the associated procedure code, rather it defines some exceptional situation surrounding the use of that code. There are approximately 300 HPCPS level 1 and 2 modifiers. For the purposes of the RBRVS, these modifiers are broken down into two primary categories: those that affect reimbursement and those that don't. Modifiers that affect reimbursement can do so resulting in either an increase or a decrease based upon the definition and use of that modifier. For example, the modifier that defines the use of multiple procedures beyond the initial primary procedure is assigned the modifier 51. By regulation, codes assigned modifier 51 will have their reimbursement reduced by 50 percent. On the other hand, modifier 50, which is used to define a procedure that is performed bilaterally when normally it would be performed on only one side, results

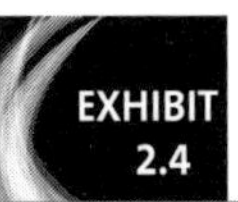

Calculating the Medicare Fee Schedule (MFS) Amount

HCPCS Code	Work RVU	Adjusted Non-Facility RVU	Adjusted Facility RVU	Non-Facility MFS	Facility MFS
10040	1.18	1.727	1.431	$58.78	$48.72
10060	1.17	1.794	1.486	$61.05	$50.59
10061	2.40	3.316	2.905	$112.88	$98.87
10080	1.17	1.984	1.525	$67.52	$51.91
10081	2.45	3.954	3.280	$134.57	$111.63
10120	1.22	1.964	1.559	$66.85	$53.08
10121	2.69	4.087	3.472	$139.12	$118.19
10140	1.53	2.200	1.909	$74.88	$64.98
10160	1.20	1.826	1.523	$62.16	$51.85
10180	2.25	3.462	3.450	$117.82	$117.42

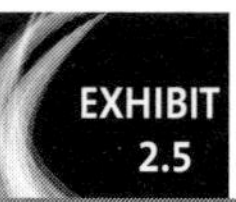
EXHIBIT 2.5

Example of Adjustment Factors for Specific Modifiers

Modifier	Factor
21	1.25
22	1.20
26	0.40
50	0.25
51	0.62
52	0.80
54	1.50
55	0.70
56	0.20
60	0.50
62	0.60
73	1.50
74	0.60
78	0.85
80	0.25
81	0.10
82	0.15
AS	0.75
FY	1.10
QB	0.25
TC	0.70

Failure to adjust the relative value unit based on the modifier factor could result in understating a physician's earning potential or productivity. It could also result in an inaccurate estimate of the practice's cost per relative value unit .

in an increase in reimbursement of 50 percent, or to 150 percent of the global fee.

Exhibit 2.5 contains a sampling of modifiers that result in an adjustment to the reimbursement along with their mathematical factors.

Although Exhibit 2.5 does not provide an exhaustive list, it does contain the utilization modifiers. In addition, some of the factors may not apply to specific practice situations and others are estimates that may be affected by other rules, such as set relationships in the RBRVS database. For example, modifiers 54, 55, and 56 describe different elements of the global surgical procedure. Modifier 54 is used to report the procedure itself, modifier 55 is used to report the presurgical element, and modifier 56 is used to report the postsurgical element. In the RBRVS database, each modifier, where present and appropriate, is assigned a fixed value, the sum of which equals 1, or 100 percent. The same holds true for modifier 26 and Technical Component (TC) modifiers, as long as they appear in the official database. The factors listed in Exhibit 2.5 for those modifiers are simply estimates based on averages. However, the remainder are based on commonly accepted reimbursement methodologies and may be changed based upon the practice's experience.

The process of adjusting RVU values by the modifier factor introduces another level of complexity in the RBRVS analysis; however, these adjustments are very important in order to represent the values accurately. Let's assume that a physician assists with surgical procedure 49000 (exploration of abdomen). The total unadjusted RVU for this procedure (for 2012) is 22.51, which equates to a geographically neutral amount for a participating provider of $766.19. When modifier 80 (assistant surgeon) is applied, the Medicare payment goes down to $122.59 because the modifier 80 pays at a rate of approximately 16 percent of the fee for the global surgical procedure. When this happens, the 64-thousand-dollar question centers around whether the RVU should also be adjusted; this really depends on what side of the compensation fence you are sitting. From the physician's perspective, the amount of time spent in the operating room is similar to the amount of time spent by the primary surgeon, so it seems unreasonable to reduce the payment by 84 percent. From the employer's perspective, it seems unreasonable to pay the assistant surgeon the same as the primary surgeon when the revenue the assistant surgeon generates is only 16 percent of that for the primary surgeon. It really creates a bit of a pickle. At the outset, when looking at adjusting the RVU value, I would definitely dump the practice expense component because the presence of another surgeon in the room doesn't add to the hard costs of the procedure. In reality, the only component at risk is the work RVU, and how that is factored is dependent upon the issue discussed above. Look at it this way. As it stands, the primary surgeon generates $61.10 per work RVU (using a work RVU value of 12.54). If you don't adjust the RVU value for the assistant surgeon, you report her revenue as $9.78 per work RVU. My experience is that this creates a bit of a problem for the physician when compensation is tied to revenue per work RVU. If you adjust the work RVU to 2.01 (16 percent of 12.54), then the assistant reports revenue that is about the same as the surgeon, creating a bit of a stir from the compensator's position.

The point is that there is no definitive answer when competing interests are involved. From a purely nonbiased perspective, it would make sense to dump the practice expense component and leave the work RVU close to the global amount because, although the risk may not be as great, the assistant surgeon still spent the same amount of time and (mostly) effort as the primary surgeon. If it's not done this way in work RVU-based compensation models, why would a physician want to work as an assistant when he or she could earn five times as much as the primary surgeon?

For procedures associated with modifiers that do not affect the level of reimbursement, such as modifiers 24 and 25, use the total RVU for the global nonmodified counterpart.

A common issue in productivity is determining the level of illness of each provider's patients.

COHEN ACUITY FACTOR

For hospitals and inpatient facilities, the advent of the diagnosis-related group (DRG) model allowed for the development of case mix calculations and comparisons. This enabled the facility to assess a severity index based upon the DRG code assigned to the case, thereby allowing relative comparisons of overall productivity and efficiency based upon the severity of the treatment protocol. Until now, providers of outpatient medical services have not had this opportunity. In the hospital setting, the entire patient experience can be captured and applied to this model, thereby allowing for development of a severity index that defines the patients' conditions. For the outpatient setting, however, the provider only captures what he or she provides to the patient and not all services and procedures that may be involved in the total care for that patient's condition. Therefore, in developing this outpatient severity index, you measure the complexity of the services provided to the patient population by the practice and not the overall condition of the patients themselves.

Relative value units measure consumption of resources, and this measurement equates to the relative complexity of the procedure. So by calculating the number of relative value units per procedure, you can estimate the relative complexity of treating a patient population.

The Cohen acuity factor (CAF), as it is represented here, can be measured using RVUs because it is assumed that RVUs measure the consumption of resources for a specific procedure or service. The overall complexity of a patient encounter can be measured by the number of management options, amount of information to be obtained during the history and physical exam, the complexity of the decision-making process, and the overall complexity of the therapeutic and/or diagnostic services. The greater this overall complexity of diagnoses and treatment, the higher the RVU value. At least this is what happens most of the time. Higher RVU values also indicate a greater risk to the provider and the patient, hence the relationship to a higher CAF.

Using this assumption, you can look at the ratio of RVUs for each procedure or service and compare this with other providers within the group

Because the Cohen acuity factor is dependent upon relative value units and relative value units are assigned based on coding, bad coding will result in inaccurate Cohen acuity factor values. It is important to validate the coding through chart reviews in order to increase the level of confidence in the Cohen acuity factor.

or against other data sets (i.e., Medicare) and get a fair comparison of the acuity level of any given value against another using the same methodology. For example, you can see that cardiac surgery has the highest overall total acuity factor of 11.661 and that allergy/immunology has the lowest rating of 0.375. This would indicate that the complexity of the services and procedures provided to the patient population for cardiac surgery, that is, the overall time, effort, risk, and expense, is approximately 35 times greater than the overall complexity of services and procedures provided to the patient population for the allergy/immunology provider.

One issue that arises when calculating the CAF is that poor coding can drive the value, giving us a skewed result. This is particularly true as it applies to E/M codes. Coding for E/M services is based upon a complex set of guidelines that, in some cases, require several hundred decisions that the provider needs to consider. Contrast this with a procedural code, such as removal of gallbladder (47620), that is usually well defined and very specific. Depending upon the influence that E/M codes have on the practice (utilization as a percent of total procedures), improper E/M coding may significantly skew what would have otherwise been an accurate understanding of the application for this model. For example, a physician who undercodes on E/M codes would have an acuity factor that would indicate that his or her patients had a lower medical need than what is otherwise the case. Overcoding, on the other hand, might indicate a higher overall level of medical complexity among the patient population than is the case. Therefore, if there is a suspicion of significant E/M coding problems, consideration should be given to resolving those issues first and then calculating the acuity factor. In many cases, a simple chart audit followed by an extrapolation calculation is all that is needed to deal with this issue. A better idea would be to break out the CAF by E/M and non-E/M services, as discussed next.

Development Assumptions

As mentioned earlier, the acuity factor is calculated based upon the RBRVS database. In order to proceed, one needs to accept the assumption that this is a valid model. The second assumption is that the RBRVS accurately measures the consumption of resources and contribution of the physician's time and effort when providing the service as assigned. This means that one must accept that the higher the RVU, the greater the consumption of resources and the greater the relative complexity of the diagnosis and treatment of the patient(s). The other assumptions are more practice/provider specific. In order to accurately measure the RVU values for the procedures, the practice must be able to accurately track both procedures and annual frequency for those procedures by provider and/or specialty. And because the procedures identified are based upon the codes selected, one must assume that the coding is accurate (or approximately accurate) with respect to the procedures actually performed and the documentation recorded in the patient's chart.

In building the database for calculating acuity, include only those procedures that have an associated official or extrapolated relative value unit value.

Calculating the Acuity Ratio

The first step in calculating the acuity ratio is to assign an RVU value to each procedure code/modifier group. Include in the table only those groups that have associated RVUs. In assigning RVU values to procedure code/modifier combinations, use the modifier-factored calculations as discussed above.

Next, take the RVU values, multiply by the frequency for that line item, and determine the sum of the products. Then sum up the total frequencies and divide the frequency into the sum total RVU amount and you end up with a ratio of RVUs to procedures.

Exhibit 2.6 shows a sample of an acuity calculation table. In this case, multiply the modifier-factored, geographically adjusted non-facility total RVU times the frequency. You then have the sum of the frequencies (448) and the sum of the total RVUs (934.81). Next, divide the total RVUs by the total frequency (934.81/448). The result, 2.087, is the total CAF for this practice, specialty, or provider.

As a process of normalizing data from the national Medicare database, you would now compare this CAF for the practice to the national Medicare average CAF for the same specialty. For cardiovascular disease, the national Medicare CAF is 1.752. Compared to the practice, the variance would be approximately 19 percent, meaning that the overall complexity of the procedures performed by this practice on their patient population is approximately 19 percent greater than the average Medicare population (assuming their specialty is cardiovascular disease). If this were a urology specialty, you would compare the CAF with that of urology (3.165), resulting in a variance of –34 percent, indicating that the complexity of the procedures the practice provides for their patient population is, on average, about a third less than that of the national Medicare patient population.

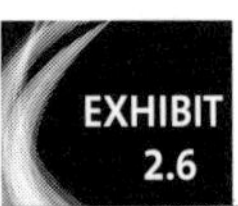

EXHIBIT 2.6 Sample Acuity Calculations

Procedure Code	Modifier	Description	Annualized Frequency	Factored Adjusted Non-Facility RVU	Total RVUs
19240	58	Removal of breast	1	30.59	30.59
19240	78	Removal of breast	4	30.59	122.38
20200	51	Muscle biopsy	4	2.68	10.70
20200		Muscle biopsy	8	5.35	42.80
20520		Removal of foreign body	1	4.83	4.83
20550	51	Inj tendon sheath/ligament	1	0.86	0.86
20550	59	Inj tendon sheath/ligament	7	1.72	12.05
20550	LT	Inj tendon sheath/ligament	15	1.72	25.82
20550	RT	Inj tendon sheath/ligament	11	1.72	18.93
20550		Inj tendon sheath/ligament	218	1.72	375.24
20551	59	Inj tendon origin/insertion	1	1.69	1.69
20551		Inj tendon origin/insertion	23	1.69	38.87
20552	RT	Inj trigger point, 1/2 muscl	1	1.65	1.65
20552		Inj trigger point, 1/2 muscl	106	1.65	174.71
20553		Inject trigger points, =/> 3	2	1.86	3.71
20600	LT	Drain/inject, joint/bursa	7	1.55	10.88
20600		Drain/inject, joint/bursa	38	1.55	59.08
		TOTALS	448		934.81

In medicine, age and sex have a great deal to do with the types and frequency of procedures and services that are provided to patients. The Medicare population is older than the general population and consists of a higher percentage of females than the general population, giving this group some unique actuarial characteristics. The importance of this calculation becomes clear in these examples; unless the practice is 100 percent Medicare, the value of the national Medicare data set is diminished to the degree that the practice's payer mix is other than Medicare, although not in some 1-to-1 linear fashion. The CAF can be used to normalize this national database for the practice by adjusting the results for their particular patient population. As you will discover later, this can be of particular importance when analyzing E/M utilization and physician productivity.

Evaluation and Management vs. Non-Evaluation and Management

One important application for the acuity factor is for rapid identification of potential E/M coding problems within the practice. As mentioned earlier, poor E/M coding has the potential to skew the overall acuity factor because of the influence that E/M codes have in most practices. Separation of E/M codes from the other groups also helps to identify utilization issues based upon comparison to the national averages by specialty.

Coding for a single E/M visit is far more complex than coding for a sophisticated procedure such as a coronary artery bypass graft. The E/M visit is not more complex than the cardiac procedure, rather the coding algorithm is far more complex. As a result, supported by study after study, improper coding for the E/M visit is more of a rule than an exception. In fact, based on three national studies conducted over the past several years, it is estimated that, given a room of 100 professional coders and a patient chart, 42 coders would disagree with the other 58 on the specific E/M code to be reported. Because of this, it is not uncommon for the total acuity factor to be skewed toward the E/M coding anomalies found within the practice. And the higher the number of E/M codes as a percent of all procedures, the greater the potential for skewing. For example, cardiac surgery providers report the highest level of both E/M and non-E/M acuity factors. This would indicate that not only are the procedures they perform extremely complex but the E/M services for those patients also indicate a higher degree of complexity. However, the ratio between non-E/M and E/M factors is 0.14, indicating that the procedures themselves are significantly more complex than the related E/M services. In pediatrics, you see an E/M acuity factor of 1.75 and a non-E/M factor of 0.70, indicating that the process of E/M for a particular patient population is less intense (or complex) than the procedures that are performed for that same patient population.

Work vs. Total Relative Value Units

E/M and non-E/M acuity measurements are also broken out by work and total RVU values in order to ensure a more specific examination of issues in both E/M utilization and physician productivity analyses. By doing so, you can further differentiate the physician work product from the actual and estimated expenses associated with the specific procedure or service. In assessing the impact here, you would expect that the work E/M acuity factor would be less than the total E/M acuity factor because the former does not consider the resources required in the form of fixed and variable expenses. However, the ratio of these two is also useful as a comparison when identifying potential E/M coding anomalies because, again, coding for non-E/M procedures is far more straightforward and less complex. This same assumption would apply to the relationship between the work non-E/M and the work E/M ratios, except that with the exclusion of resources other than those measured by the work RVU, you have a more accurate process for measuring the physician's contribution to productivity.

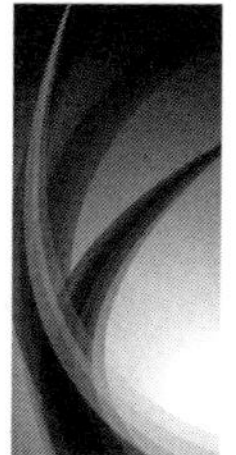

CHAPTER 3

Understanding Conversion Factors

Many in the healthcare industry believe that the conversion factor is a value dictated by Congress and the Centers for Medicare & Medicaid Services. Although this is true for Medicare, it is not true for other fee schedules used by the practice or by payers. Understanding the fundamentals of how to calculate, interpret, and apply the concept of the conversion factor will allow the practice to better understand its financial targets.

WHAT IS THE CONVERSION FACTOR?

The conversion factor (CF) is a value that is used to convert the relative value unit (RVU) amount into a usable format, specifically the fee. With Medicare, for example, you are given the CF as the Congress mandates it to the Centers for Medicare & Medicaid Services (CMS). Multiplied by the total geographically adjusted RVU, it determines what the practice is allowed when treating a Medicare patient. In most practices, however, the fee schedule has evolved over time, through the use of methods other than the Medicare fee schedule. Therefore, in these practices, each procedure code will have a unique CF: unique in the sense that the fee divided by the total adjusted RVU will be different for all procedure codes used. The exception here is when the fee schedule for the practice is developed using the resource-based relative value scale (RBRVS) or as a percent of Medicare. In those cases, because Medicare is directly related to the RBRVS, the CF values for the practice would mirror those for Medicare.

The conversion factor is a dollar value used to convert the relative value unit to a fee. It is also used as a relative measurement of the practice's fee schedule to determine variances within specific coding groups.

Another issue of some importance is the division of codes into major categories for the development of CF calculations. The RBRVS is developed for all procedure codes and code categories using the same methodology.

This means that whether the code is an office visit code or a code for open-heart surgery, the methodology for assigning the values to each of the components is consistent, at least in theory. Implementation issues arise when this is applied to the real world and competitive market forces come into play. For example, patients call several offices to price-shop office visit fees. However, it is unusual for a patient to call a practice to shop the fee for an appendectomy or for a complex surgical procedure. As a result, the CF levels (i.e., the charge per RVU) for some code categories, such as evaluation and management (E/M), are much lower than for surgery. So when calculating CF levels for the practice, consider doing so by major code category, as follows:

When doing conversion factor calculations, it is important to break the practice down into major coding groups to allow for competitive market acceptance.

Surgery	10000–69999
Radiology	70000–79999
Pathology and lab	80000–89999
Medicine	90000–99999 (excluding 99201–99499)
E/M	99201–99499
Health Care Financing Administration Current Procedural Coding System (HCPCS) II	A0000–X9999

Some specialty practices will have experience with the subdivisions found within Current Procedural Terminology (CPT). For example, within surgery, there are sections for the integumentary, musculoskeletal, respiratory, cardiovascular, digestive, gastroenterology, endocrine, and neurology systems, to name a few. Within these subdivisions are even more divisions, each with greater specificity. The specialty practice will have (or should have) experience with its own subsections of CPT and, as such, may break out the CF calculations differently. Remember that if you go below nine data points, it will be more difficult for you to obtain meaningful calculations.

The reasons for divisional calculations will become clearer as you proceed through the rest of this chapter.

The conversion factor can be used to determine viability of managed care contracts, pricing and charge profiles, establishment of fees for new procedures, and similar factors.

HOW IS THE CONVERSION FACTOR USED?

You have seen the application for Medicare—to calculate the payment for a procedure billed to Medicare. There are, however, many other uses for the CF. For example, you can divide the fee schedule into coding categories, such as surgery, radiology, pathology, medicine, and E/M. These can be further broken down into subcategories. Then, by applying the formula that appears in the section below (Calculating the Conversion Factor), you can calculate the CF for each division. This is important in understanding how to profile the fee schedule and apply this to various market and competitive factors and also for establishing new fees for new procedures or adjusting aberrant fees for existing procedures.

If you know the relative value unit amount (it is published) and your fee, you can determine the conversion factor for each code by dividing the relative value unit into the fee.

CALCULATING THE CONVERSION FACTOR

Basic algebra assumes that if you have three variables and you know two of them, you can easily solve for the third. In this application, having the RVU amounts and the fees, you can easily calculate the CF by dividing the fee by the RVU, as follows:

$691.10/14.197 = 48.6793

A problem arises, however, when there is more than one CF to calculate in order to obtain the CF for an entire charge profile or even a group of codes. Next, you will explore two methods for determining the average CF for a set of procedure codes.

WEIGHTED VS. LINEAR AVERAGE

A straight, or linear, average looks only at the total divided by the number in the sample. A weighted average gives value to the frequency of occurrence.

To determine an average amount for any set of numbers, simply add the numbers together and divide the sum by the number of records (or examples) in your data set. For example, if you add the following seven numbers:

10, 12, 10, 22, 30, 14, 16,

you get a sum of 114. If you divide that sum by the number of records (7), you get a mathematical average of 16.29. In some cases, however, each number may be represented by a frequency, which identifies the number of times that particular number would appear in the records. Giving consideration to this volume of occurrences is referred to as weighting the average. In a weighted average, you give weight, or additional consideration, to a value based upon the number of times it appears in the database, or its frequency of occurrence.

The straight average conversion factor is simple to obtain. Just determine the conversion factor for each procedure, add them together, and then divide the total by the number of records in the data set.

Calculating the Average Conversion Factor

To determine the average CF, simply add the sum of the values for the CF for each code and then divide by the number of codes in the data set. Exhibit 3.1 contains the fee, RVU, and CF for seven surgical procedure codes.

To get the CF for each code, divide the RVU for that procedure into the fee. For example, the fee for code 1 is $1,087 and the RVU is equal to 10.215. If you divide 10.215 into the fee of $1,087, it equals 106.42, which is the CF for that code. This means that the charge for this procedure code is equal to $106.42 for each RVU assigned to that code.

To obtain the mathematical average for the CF, determine the sum for all seven CFs listed and divide this by the number of records, as follows:

$$652.79/7 = 93.26$$

The problem with using a straight average is that it gives as much weight to codes that have poorly managed fees as it does to those that have well-managed fees.

Notice that there is quite a variance between the CF levels for different codes within the same major category. The wide variance indicates that there is a lack of consistency in the fee scheduling methodology or it points to methodologies other than the use of Medicare or RBRVS. This is one reason why the straight average is not a good representation of the practice's fee scheduling process. Experience shows that the codes for procedures that are performed most frequently get the most attention. The problem is that by using a straight average, codes that are not managed well have an equal influence on the final value. You run into problems when you attempt to apply that final value to other analysis models.

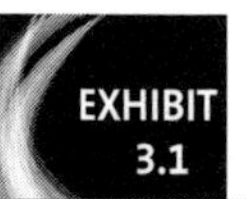

Average Conversion Factor Calculation

Code	Fee	RVU	CF
Code 1	$1,087	10.215	106.42
Code 2	$365	5.343	68.31
Code 3	$1,114	13.713	81.24
Code 4	$2,487	14.051	177.65
Code 5	$529	6.185	85.53
Code 6	$887	14.222	63.37
Code 7	$996	14.173	70.27
TOTAL			652.79

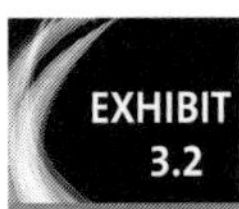

EXHIBIT 3.2

Calculating the Weighted Average Conversion Factor

Code	Fee	RVU	Freq	Total Fee	Total RVU	CF
Code 1	$1,087	10.215	1	$1,087	10.215	106.42
Code 2	$365	5.343	7	$2,555	37.401	68.31
Code 3	$1,114	13.713	12	$13,368	164.556	81.24
Code 4	$2,487	14.051	1	$2,487	14.051	177.65
Code 5	$529	6.185	12	$6,348	74.220	85.53
Code 6	$887	14.222	60	$53,220	853.320	63.37
Code 7	$996	14.173	108	$107,568	1,530.684	70.27
TOTALS				$186,633	2,684.447	652.79

Calculating the Weighted Average Conversion Factor

In order to balance the consideration given to those procedures that are performed the most, it is important to "weight" the average based upon annual frequency. Again, the assumption is that fees for high-volume procedures are better managed than those performed once, twice, or only a few times. In this case, it is necessary to have the annual frequency for each procedure code.

Using the weighted average, assign the value of a particular code to determine the average conversion factor based upon its contribution to the fee schedule as a whole.

In Exhibit 3.2 the Total Fee column represents the Fee column multiplied by the Frequency column. The Total RVU column represents the RVU column multiplied by the Frequency column.

Note that whether you divide the RVU into the Fee or the Total RVU into the Total Fee, the individual CF remains the same. The difference occurs when you solve for the sum of the products of the Total Fees and the Total RVUs.

First, determine the sum of the Total Fees, which is $186,633.

Then determine the sum of the Total RVUs, which is 2,684.447.

Finally, divide the Total Fees by the Total RVUs, as follows:

$186,633/2,684.447 = $69.52

The value of $69.52 is the average CF when weighted for the frequency of the procedures that were performed. This method is recommended if, in fact, the frequencies are available from the practice.

Using either the total RVU and total fees or individual RVUs and individual fees, the individual conversion factor remains the same.

Note that dividing the frequency-adjusted RVU into the frequency-adjusted fee renders the same individual CF as in the previous example.

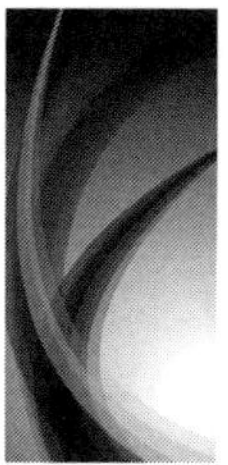

CHAPTER 4

Procedural Cost Accounting

Fewer than 6 percent of medical practices have any clue as to what the hard costs are for the products they sell. Knowing the actual cost of delivering a service or performing a procedure is not only valuable but also necessary for survival in an intensely competitive marketplace. No other industry could have survived as long as the healthcare industry with the lack of financial accountability that it has shown.

Since the introduction of managed care concepts, physicians have been outmaneuvered by the insurance carriers' ability to dance around the issue of cost with relation to fixed fee schedules. In the past, the physician had to engage in expensive and intrusive processes in order to calculate what it cost to perform a particular procedure and whether the proposed managed care fee schedule was fair to the bottom line. Many practices, when faced with the possibility of a large managed care contract, spend thousands of dollars on legal fees to ensure the wording is correct; however, they don't take the time to first determine whether the contract is profitable.

Knowledge of the actual cost for each procedure performed or service provided is crucial for establishing a profitable fee schedule.

With a cost and profit/loss analysis, you can develop a database that will provide you with the information necessary to perform a true and cost-effective assessment of your financial condition. And as a bonus, much of the data will serve as an internal benchmark for measuring the success of financially related processes, such as billing, collections, and cost containment efforts.

This information is very powerful when it comes to preparing the practice for managed care negotiations. Knowing what the break-even fee is for each procedure based upon resource-based relative value scale

The resource-based relative value scale is here to stay, and the sooner you become knowledgeable on the methodology, the sooner you can apply it to your advantage.

(RBRVS) costing techniques provides a justifiable and standardized method that the practice can use to defend its position on individual fee amounts.

The cost accounting analysis also identifies consistency levels for the comparison of one proced ure code to another. This process allows the practice to compare its collection rate to its expense rate. It can be used to determine, by procedure code, whether the practice is making or losing money and how much profit or loss there is by unit and by year. If properly tracked, this information can also help practices to measure their cost ratios on a month-to-month basis for comparison with financial goals and budgets.

The fact is the RBRVS is here to stay. More and more managed care providers will depend upon the RBRVS to either negotiate fee schedules or determine reasonable practice costs. These factors are more significant when there is a high managed care mix within the practice. This will be supported through the ability to track and manage practice costs and fee levels and to benchmark the practice using the RBRVS database.

By breaking the cost analysis down to the lowest level, you can begin to micromanage your practice's financial processes.

Cost accounting techniques take on a number of different forms. In fact, entire books have been written on the topic. Cost accounting can be studied at the financial level, the managerial level, the applications level, and so on. Our focus is on its relationship to the revenue base of the practice, line-item procedural relationships, and overall costing of procedures and services. The point is to concentrate on using the RBRVS as a tool to compare utilization levels, resource allocation, profit and loss levels, common costing, and other bits of critical information for the practice. Study this from both a macro level (e.g., global amounts such as total billing and collections) and on a micro level (per procedure and per unit comparisons). After completing the data collection and analysis portion, examine some practical applications for cost accounting analyses.

To start the analysis, you need to be able to identify the commercial fee for each procedure as well as the number of times per year the procedure is performed.

DATA REQUIREMENTS FOR COST ACCOUNTING

The following data are required for each procedure code/modifier combination:

- Annual frequency
- RBRVS individual relative value unit (RVU; geographically adjusted)
- Total RBRVS units
- Total billed amount

The following data are required for the practice:

- Total RBRVS units
- Total practice expense
  - Broken out by category (fixed, variable, etc.)
  - With and without physician compensation/distribution
- Average collection as a percent of gross charges
  - Either for the practice as a whole or by procedure code/modifier group

Because this is an analysis based on the resource-based relative value scale, it is necessary to be able to associate the relative value unit components with each procedure code.

To begin this analysis, develop a complete fee schedule, including both the fee charged and the annual (or period) frequency for each procedure. You also need a complete listing of each RVU component contained within the RBRVS for each procedure code and the geographic adjustment factor (GAF) amounts for each component. Then obtain the practice's collections as a percent of gross billing and its costs as a percent of gross billings. An entire volume can be written with respect to the latter, depending upon the final use for the cost accounting data set. For example, if you are looking to negotiate a managed care contract, you may want to include only a reasonable salary for the physician. If you are looking to determine the profitability of a capitation contract, you may want to include only the variable expenses. If you are looking to make an internal cost comparison with respect to other ventures or to other departments, you may want to exclude all or part of the physician compensation package. You can change the assumptions as needed to perform what-if analyses.

A WORD ABOUT PRACTICE EXPENSE

You must assume that each procedure code has a cost that is relative to the other procedure codes based upon the relative value unit values assigned.

One downfall of using an established data set like the RBRVS is that not every procedure code has RVU values. This means that you may not be able to include every code in the analysis database. For example, many of the pathology/laboratory codes (80000–89999) do not have established RVUs, excluding them from the spreadsheet. The problem is that there may be a substantial cost associated with these procedures, and, if the revenue is not also excluded, the analysis may become skewed. One reason for using the cost as a percent of the gross billing is that it allows you to assume that the total practice costs are at least somewhat evenly distributed across all service categories. Then you can apply that percent to the total billing amount reported only among those procedures that have

It is common to find that not all procedure codes the practice delivers have relative value unit values. This is why a percent of expenses to gross charges is used and applied to the table that contains the codes that do have relative value unit values.

Don't forget to exclude those codes that have variable expense amounts from the table, for example, supplies and drugs.

The three main expense categories are fixed, variable, and direct. It is important to understand how these are defined in your practice.

an associated RVU. While still excluding those procedures without RVUs from the analysis, this method ensures that those included are represented accurately and therefore the results will also be accurate.

For example, if a practice has $1,000,000 in gross charges and the total calculated expenses equal $500,000, you would calculate the cost at 50 percent of the gross billing. This is important because you then assume that each procedure code costs about 50 percent of the actual value to deliver. Although this may not be true on a line-item basis, the assumption is important in order to calculate the total values. If, in the example, $150,000 worth of procedure codes (and frequencies) is not included in the sample set because the codes lack RVU values, only $850,000 of the total revenue generated would be represented in your table. If you divided the expense value of $500,000 into that $850,000 in represented charges, your expense percent would jump to 58.8 percent, an inaccurate assumption. In order to maintain the integrity of the relationship of expense to each code, you would multiply the $850,000 by 50 percent and come up with a cost for providing the represented services and procedures of $425,000. In other words, although it costs $500,000 to generate $1,000,000 in charges, it, respectively, costs $425,000 to generate $850,000 in charges.

The other issue involving exclusion of codes from the database has to do with procedure codes that represent services with variable costs (i.e., certain modified procedures) or those that are directly related to the cost of the product represented by the code, such as supply codes (99070 and alphanumeric Health Care Financing Administration Current Procedural Coding System [HCPCS] codes) and drug codes (HCPCS Level 2 J codes). For the most part, these codes are priced based upon either regulatory models (for Medicare and other Title XIX programs) or by a cost-plus-markup methodology. They therefore have a direct relationship to costs that are independent from the RBRVS model. Administration of some of these codes also involves a practice expense, but this is usually reported using an associated code such as a 90788 (injection of an antibiotic).

A WORD ABOUT EXPENSE CATEGORIES

There are several ways to determine expenses, and it is important to involve the practice's certified public accountant or financial manager in this process. When the cost analysis is performed, expenses are broken down into four categories:

- *Fixed expenses,* which include staff salaries, lease payments, rent, utilities, etc.
- *Variable expenses,* which include those expenses directly linked to patient visit and volume, such as surgical kits, table paper, charts, gowns, etc.
- *Direct expenses,* which represent expenses that are directly attributable to a specific provider. This might include malpractice insurance, a leased vehicle, or specialized medical staff.
- *Owner compensation,* which normally includes those compensation expenses above a reasonable salary for the physician and other owners of the corporation and bonuses distributed to both owners and nonowners.

By relating the different expense categories to the associated relative value unit components, you can more accurately define those areas that affect the practice's overall profitability.

APPLICATION OF EXPENSE CATEGORIES

The RVU component(s) used for the cost calculations will be dependent upon the expense category(ies) selected. When looking at the big picture of the practice, you normally include all expense categories and use the total adjusted RVU values. When looking at operational and infrastructure expense issues, you normally use only the fixed and variable expenses and relate them to the practice and malpractice expense RVU values. When looking only at the effect of physician compensation issues, you use the physician compensation and bonus expenses and relate them to the work RVU value only. Direct expenses are sometimes factored into this latter category when developing provider-based cost centers for compensation consideration.

By breaking the results down into analytical categories, you can address several different applications for the results.

COST ACCOUNTING RESULTS

When you apply these principles and models, your goal is to determine the following for each procedure code:

- Performance cost (or the cost of actually delivering the service)
- Average collection (or actual, if that information is available)
- Profit or loss
- Break-even fee amount

Any spreadsheet program will work. If you are familiar with a relational program, such as Power Builder or Access, it will be easier to build some of the tables using relational techniques.

For the entire practice or group as a whole, your goal is to determine:

- Total resource utilization for all codes
- Cost per unit (RVU)
- Profit or loss per unit and for the entire control group

BUILDING THE SPREADSHEET

First you will need to set up a spreadsheet on your computer or use a graph ledger (Exhibit 4.1). In the first few columns, put the procedure code with modifier, if any; the fee amount; the annual frequency; the adjusted RVU; the total fee amount; the total RVUs; the Medicare fee schedule (MFS) amount; and the conversion factor (CF).

This is the same spreadsheet you built in Chapter 2, so it is not necessary to reenter the data for a cost accounting analysis.

Excel spreadsheet templates, which are on the companion CD-ROM, will assist you in building these tables.

Total Adjusted Relative Value Unit

To calculate total adjusted RVU, use the RBRVS calculations as discussed above. If you decide to go with the actual adjusted RVU, as is used in the Medicare calculations, you will be able to use the actual MFS. If not, the MFS column can be labeled differently.

Total Relative Value Units per Procedure (TOT RVU)

Multiply the total geographically adjusted RVU for each procedure by the annual frequency. This will give you the total annual utilization.

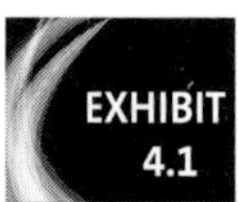
EXHIBIT 4.1 Building the Basic Cost Accounting Table

Code	Fee	Freq	RVU	Tot Fee	Tot RVU	MFS	CF
10040	$102	61	1.783	$6,222	108.73	$64.53	57.31
10060	$145	191	1.850	$27,695	353.35	$66.97	78.38
10061	$199	58	3.415	$11,542	198.07	$123.62	58.27
10080	$117	270	2.048	$31,590	552.83	$74.12	57.31
10081	$101	208	4.060	$21,008	844.48	$146.97	24.88
10120	$116	66	2.025	$7,656	133.65	$73.30	57.31
10121	$224	144	4.208	$32,256	605.88	$152.31	53.24
10140	$55	89	2.265	$4,895	201.59	$81.99	24.28
10160	$108	142	1.880	$15,336	266.96	$68.05	57.31
10180	$194	336	3.543	$65,184	1190.28	$128.24	54.76

Total Billed per Procedure

Next, multiply the commercial fee amount by the annual frequency to get the total billed per procedure.

Medicare Fee Schedule Amount

Multiply the Medicare CF by the adjusted RVU amount to get the MFS equivalent amount. If you decide to go with the actual adjusted RVU, as is used in the Medicare calculations, you will be able to use the actual MFS. If not, the MFS column can be labeled differently. In any case, because of minor variations in methodologies permitted from carrier to carrier, this number may or may not be exactly equal to the MFS, but it should be very close.

Practice-Specific Conversion Factor

Divide the adjusted RVU into the fee to get the current CF for that code.

Once all basic data have been entered, calculate the totals at the bottom of the applicable columns.

Totaling Fees and Relative Value Units

The next step is to determine the line-item totals for the fees and the RVUs (Exhibit 4.2).

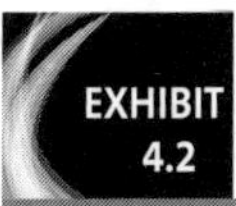
EXHIBIT 4.2 Getting Grand Totals for Fees and Relative Value Units

Code	Fee	Freq	RVU	Tot Fee	Tot RVU	MFS	CF
10040	$102	61	1.783	$6,222	108.73	$64.53	57.31
10060	$145	191	1.850	$27,695	353.35	$66.97	78.38
10061	$199	58	3.415	$11,542	198.07	$123.62	58.27
10080	$117	270	2.048	$31,590	552.83	$74.12	57.31
10081	$101	208	4.060	$21,008	844.48	$146.97	24.88
10120	$116	66	2.025	$7,656	133.65	$73.30	57.31
10121	$224	144	4.208	$32,256	605.88	$152.31	53.24
10140	$55	89	2.265	$4,895	201.59	$81.99	24.28
10160	$108	142	1.880	$15,336	266.96	$68.05	57.31
10180	$194	336	3.543	$65,184	1190.28	$128.24	54.76
	TOTALS			$223,384	4455.81		

Total Billed for the Fee Schedule

At the bottom of the total billed (Tot Fee) column, add up all procedure codes to get the total billed amount for the fee schedule.

Total Relative Value Unit for the Fee Schedule

Next, total all of the procedural RVUs to get the total RVU for the fee schedule.

Remember, you are basing this on the applicable expense amount divided by the calculated gross charges.

► Calculating Expense Percent

Here you apply the concept discussed above concerning the determination of prospective costs based upon the actual expense percent of the gross charges. Take the commercial fee times the frequency to get the total calculated charges. Then, divide the total expense amount by the total calculated charges. Multiply that same expense percent by the total gross charges within the sample set. This will equal the cost of generating the charges for those services contained within the sample set.

Example of Expense Percent

The expense percent for the entire practice is applied to the table of codes that have relative value unit values.

Multiply the expense percent for the practice by the total charges calculated in the table. Then, divide this by the sum total relative value units to obtain the cost per relative value unit.

In this example, the estimated cost of doing business for the procedures that are included in the table are calculated. Remember, only those line items with an RVU value should be used in this calculation.

- The practice generates $300,000 in charges.
- $181,897 are calculated as expenses.
- Divide expenses into gross charges
  - $181,897/$300,000 = .606 or 60.6 percent.
- $223,384 in charges are represented in the data set
  - $76,617 in procedures do not have RVU values.
- Multiply the represented charges by the expense percent to get the dollar cost for the sample set
  - $223,384 * 60.6 percent = $135,443.

► Calculating the Relative Value Unit Cost Factors

The next step is to determine the expense amount by either factoring the percent of gross billing or using the actual expense amount (Exhibit 4.3).

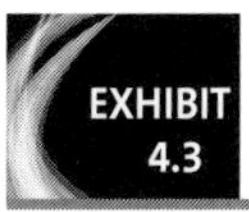

Calculating the Cost per Relative Value Unit and the Practice Conversion Factor

Code	Fee	Freq	RVU	Tot Fee	Tot RVU	MFS	CF
10040	$102	61	1.783	$6,222	108.73	$64.53	57.31
10060	$145	191	1.850	$27,695	353.35	$66.97	78.38
10061	$199	58	3.415	$11,542	198.07	$123.62	58.27
10080	$117	270	2.048	$31,590	552.83	$74.12	57.31
10081	$101	208	4.060	$21,008	844.48	$146.97	24.88
10120	$116	66	2.025	$7,656	133.65	$73.30	57.31
10121	$224	144	4.208	$32,256	605.88	$152.31	53.24
10140	$55	89	2.265	$4,895	201.59	$81.99	24.28
10160	$108	142	1.880	$15,336	266.96	$68.05	57.31
10180	$194	336	3.543	$65,184	1190.28	$128.24	54.76
TOTALS				$223,384	4455.81		
Variable Expense		**$135,443**		Cost per RVU			**30.40**

In determining this amount, you may have to consider several factors such as the physician compensation or salary package; whether to use fixed and variable or just variable marginal expenses for contracts; etc. For this example, you are using a variable expense amount of $135,443.

Total Cost

Multiply the total billed for the fee schedule by the expense percentage (or use the actual expense amount).

This calculation will identify what it costs you to provide a particular service.

Cost per Relative Value Unit

Determine the cost per RVU by dividing the cost amount for the fee schedule by the total RVUs for the fee schedule. In this case, you would divide $135,443 by 4,455.82.

Calculating the Cost per Occurrence

Go back to each line item in the spreadsheet and, in another column, multiply the procedural RVU by the cost per RVU (Exhibit 4.4). This will identify the cost for that particular procedure.

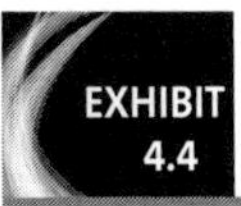

EXHIBIT 4.4

Calculating the Cost for Each Procedure Code

Code	Fee	Freq	RVU	Tot Fee	Tot RVU	MFS	CF	Cost
10040	$102	61	1.783	$6,222	108.73	$64.53	57.31	**$54.18**
10060	$145	191	1.850	$27,695	353.35	$66.97	78.38	**$56.23**
10061	$199	58	3.415	$11,542	198.07	$123.62	58.27	**$103.81**
10080	$117	270	2.048	$31,590	552.83	$74.12	57.31	**$62.24**
10081	$101	208	4.060	$21,008	844.48	$146.97	24.88	**$123.41**
10120	$116	66	2.025	$7,656	133.65	$73.30	57.31	**$61.55**
10121	$224	144	4.208	$32,256	605.88	$152.31	53.24	**$127.90**
10140	$55	89	2.265	$4,895	201.59	$81.99	24.28	**$68.85**
10160	$108	142	1.880	$15,336	266.96	$68.05	57.31	**$57.15**
10180	$194	336	3.543	$65,184	1190.28	$128.24	54.76	**$107.68**
TOTALS				$223,384	4455.81			
Expense		$135,443		Cost per RVU			30.40	

A Word about Collections

This is a great way to identify codes that need to have a serious analysis of their fees.

Normally, collection is calculated as a percent of gross charges by simply dividing the gross revenue (or collected amount during the sample period) by the gross charges. Sometimes, however, situations exist that can significantly skew this calculation. For example, if the practice engages in a first-time aggressive collection effort, it may reduce accounts receivable (A/R) by significantly increasing collections. The problem is that this increase in collections may be a one-time event and may not reflect the revenue for codes billed during the data period in which the gross charges were generated. The opposite may also occur if the practice experiences a significant increase in A/R for some reason.

Normally, you assume collections based upon total receipts divided by gross charges. If you are able to calculate the actual collection percent by procedure, then use those values instead.

The other situation that may occur is that the practice may have a management system that tracks actual or average collection by procedure code. If this is the case, then simply replace the collection amount calculated in the examples using average collections for the practice with these more accurate values.

Calculating Profit and Loss Amounts

Now that you have calculated the costs for each procedure and know the annual frequency, you can calculate the profit/loss amounts for each code and for the entire practice (Exhibit 4.5). This information is very important

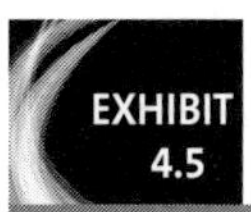

EXHIBIT 4.5 Using Average Collections to Calculate Profit and Loss Amounts

Code	Fee	MFS	Freq	RVU	CF	Tot Fee	Tot RVU	Cost Per Occurrence	Collect	P/L	Total P/L
10040	$102	$61.91	61	1.783	57.31	$6,231	108.73	$54.18	$81.72	**$27.54**	**$1,679.77**
10060	$145	$64.25	191	1.850	78.38	$27,695	353.35	$56.23	$116.00	**$59.77**	**$11,415.25**
10061	$199	$118.61	58	3.415	58.27	$11,542	198.07	$103.81	$159.20	**$55.39**	**$3,212.88**
10080	$117	$71.11	270	2.048	57.31	$31,681	552.83	$62.24	$93.87	**$31.63**	**$8,540.40**
10081	$101	$141.01	208	4.060	24.88	$21,008	844.48	$123.41	$80.80	**($42.61)**	**($8,863.20)**
10120	$116	$70.33	66	2.025	57.31	$7,659	133.65	$61.55	$92.84	**$31.28**	**$2,064.71**
10121	$224	$146.13	144	4.208	53.24	$32,256	605.88	$127.90	$179.20	**$51.30**	**$7,387.91**
10140	$55	$78.67	89	2.265	24.28	$4,895	201.59	$68.85	$44.00	**($24.85)**	**($2,211.56)**
10160	$108	$65.30	142	1.880	57.31	$15,299	266.96	$57.15	$86.19	**$29.04**	**$4,124.17**
10180	$194	$123.04	336	3.543	54.76	$65,184	1190.28	$107.68	$155.20	**$47.52**	**$15,966.35**

for determining the reasonability of both the fee schedule and service delivery.

Collection Amount (Collection)

Multiply the fee amount by the collection percentage.

Profit/Loss per Unit

Next, subtract the cost per unit from the collection per unit to determine if there is a profit or loss for each procedure.

Annual Profit/Loss per Procedure

In the next column, multiply the profit or loss for each procedure by the annual frequency for that procedure.

► Calculating Break-Even Fees

Finally, divide the cost per occurrence by the collection percent to get the break-even fee (Exhibit 4.6). This is the amount that the practice will need to bill using the current cost and collection percent amounts to cover its costs with actual receipts.

This is a great tool to use when looking at managed care contracts.

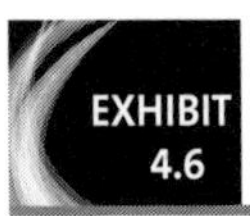

EXHIBIT 4.6

Calculating the Break-Even Fee Amount

Code	Fee	MFS	Freq	RVU	CF	Tot Fee	Tot RVU	Cost Per Occurrence	Collect	P/L	Total P/L	Break Even
10040	$102	$61.91	61	1.783	57.31	$6,231	108.73	$54.18	$81.72	$27.54	$1,679.77	**$67.73**
10060	$145	$64.25	191	1.850	78.38	$27,695	353.35	$56.23	$116.00	$59.77	$11,415.25	**$70.29**
10061	$199	$118.61	58	3.415	58.27	$11,542	198.07	$103.81	$159.20	$55.39	$3,212.88	**$129.76**
10080	$117	$71.11	270	2.048	57.31	$31,681	552.83	$62.24	$93.87	$31.63	$8,540.40	**$77.80**
10081	$101	$141.01	208	4.060	24.88	$21,008	844.48	$123.41	$80.80	($42.61)	($8,863.20)	**$154.26**
10120	$116	$70.33	66	2.025	57.31	$7,659	133.65	$61.55	$92.84	$31.28	$2,064.71	**$76.94**
10121	$224	$146.13	144	4.208	53.24	$32,256	605.88	$127.90	$179.20	$51.30	$7,387.91	**$159.87**
10140	$55	$78.67	89	2.265	24.28	$4,895	201.59	$68.85	$44.00	($24.85)	($2,211.56)	**$86.06**
10160	$108	$65.30	142	1.880	57.31	$15,299	266.96	$57.15	$86.19	$29.04	$4,124.17	**$71.43**
10180	$194	$123.04	336	3.543	54.76	$65,184	1190.28	$107.68	$155.20	$47.52	$15,966.35	**$134.60**

► Calculating Resource Allocation

The completed table can be used for a number of additional analyses. One important function is to sort the table by total RVUs (Exhibit 4.7). This is referred to as a *resource allocation table*. It allows you to see which procedures in the practice consume the greatest number of resources. When calculated by physicians and/or locations, it allows you to determine the profitability for each segment by developing production/consumption ratios.

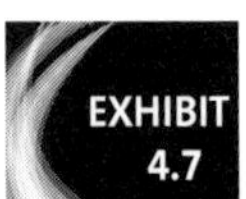

EXHIBIT 4.7

Sorting the Cost Accounting Table by Total Relative Value Units

Code	Fee	MFS	Freq	RVU	CF	Tot Fee	Tot RVU	Cost Per Occurrence	Collect	P/L	Total P/L	Break Even
10180	$194	$123.04	336	3.543	54.76	$65,184	**1190.28**	$107.68	$155.20	$47.52	$15,966.35	$134.60
10081	$101	$141.01	208	4.060	24.88	$21,008	**844.48**	$123.41	$80.80	($42.61)	($8,863.20)	$154.26
10121	$224	$146.13	144	4.208	53.24	$32,256	**605.88**	$127.90	$179.20	$51.30	$7,387.91	$159.87
10080	$117	$71.11	270	2.048	57.31	$31,681	**552.83**	$62.24	$93.87	$31.63	$8,540.40	$77.80
10060	$145	$64.25	191	1.850	78.38	$27,695	**353.35**	$56.23	$116.00	$59.77	$11,415.25	$70.29
10160	$108	$65.30	142	1.880	57.31	$15,299	**266.96**	$57.15	$86.19	$29.04	$4,124.17	$71.43
10140	$55	$78.67	89	2.265	24.28	$4,895	**201.59**	$68.85	$44.00	($24.85)	($2,211.56)	$86.06
10061	$199	$118.61	58	3.415	58.27	$11,542	**198.07**	$103.81	$159.20	$55.39	$3,212.88	$129.76
10120	$116	$70.33	66	2.025	57.31	$7,659	**133.65**	$61.55	$92.84	$31.28	$2,064.71	$76.94
10040	$102	$61.91	61	1.783	57.31	$6,231	**108.73**	$54.18	$81.72	$27.54	$1,679.77	$67.73

Notice in Exhibit 4.7 that once the values have been sorted by total RVUs, the procedure that consumes the second highest amount of resources for the practice is actually losing money each time it is performed. These types of analyses are very valuable for identifying fee schedule problems and for defending increases that are sometimes higher than you would normally expect.

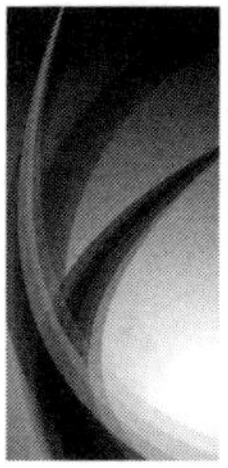

CHAPTER 5

Global Pricing and Cost Analysis

The fact is, fee-for-service just doesn't work. It creates an environment where any provider can overutilize tests, procedures, and services. On the other hand, capitation models don't work either. Not only do they encourage underutilization of necessary services and procedures but they also encourage an overutilization of physician services by the patient. It is said that in any argument, there are three sides: There is his side and her side, and somewhere in the middle is the truth.

The basic concept of global packaging involves paying the contracting entity to administer the claims as well as to manage the patient.

Several years ago, the Centers for Medicare & Medicaid Services ([CMS]; then called the Health Care Financing Administration [HCFA]) started a demonstration project using a global payment methodology. According to those involved from both the payer and provider sides, it was a success. Under this payment concept, the carrier (in this case CMS) would contract with a private entity, such as a physician–hospital organization or a hospital (only hospitals were used for the demonstration project) for a limited number of diagnosis-related groups (DRGs). CMS would then write the hospital a single check to manage all aspects of a case from hospital admission to release and discharge, including physician, hospital, and supply charges. This type of payment concept has gained much attention in the private sector, and some private carriers have already developed systems similar to the CMS program.

Writing one check for the entire episode can save the payer between 13 and 20 percent.

The most obvious benefit to the payer is that it allows the payer to control the cost of administering claims for a patient incident or episode. The cost to the payer for claims administration ranges from 13 to 20 percent of the payment amount. Under the global packaging model, the insurance company can save 75 percent or more of this expense. It also eliminates the need to pay multiple claims for the same episode on the same patient, eliminating potential over- and/or underpayment errors.

It is very important to examine this type of methodology now because it may significantly affect the way medical services are contracted and paid for in the near future. Entities that enter into these types of arrangements with carriers will approach individual medical practices to participate in bidding for case-managed groupings.

APPLICATION TO THE PHYSICIAN MARKET

Fee-for-service doesn't work. And it's no secret that prepaid plans, such as capitation, do not work either.

The bottom line is that fee-for-service does not work. It provides financial incentives for physicians to overutilize medical services and treatments, to the degree that many of those are considered medically unnecessary. On the other side, capitation-type models also do not work because they encourage an underutilization of medical services and treatments, even when such are medically necessary and reasonably available. Unfortunately, this model also encourages overutilization of physician visits by the patient, putting a tremendous financial burden on the typical medical practice.

Global models encourage a coordination of care between the physician and the patient.

One major benefit of the global package is that it encourages a coordination of care between the patient and the physician, placing control of the medical episode back where it belongs—in the physician–patient relationship. This is evidenced by the virtual elimination of precertification and preauthorization events during the treatment episode.

AMBULATORY DIAGNOSIS–RELATED GROUPS

Similar in concept to the diagnosis-related groups for hospitals, this methodology is referred to as ADRG, or ambulatory diagnosis-related groups .

A DRG is a designation assigned to individual inpatient procedures that are grouped into categories based upon certain diagnostic and treatment similarities. Hospitals have been paid based upon this methodology for many years. It appears that physicians may not be too far from this type of reimbursement, which is referred to as ambulatory DRG (ADRG) because it is managed within the scope of the physician's office as opposed to an inpatient setting.

Because practices may be called upon in the near future to competitively bid to provide specific medical services, the need to understand cost by diagnoses and treatment, or case management, is critical. Using this method and applying the cost accounting tables developed earlier, you can determine what the cost will be to treat a specific illness or injury by selecting the procedures that will be used as part of the treatment protocol.

BUILDING THE GLOBAL MODEL

Remember, this type of methodology will work only on conditions that have a definitive beginning and termination, such as an injury or acute condition. It is nearly impossible to apply this to chronic diseases and illnesses such as diabetes, chronic obstructive pulmonary disease, human immunodeficiency virus, and the like. In considering which conditions to sample, pick those for which the diagnoses and treatment protocols will be the most consistent and easily identified. There are five steps in the process of costing diagnostic categories, which are described in the following paragraphs.

Global modeling is most applicable to acute illnesses and injuries and less applicable to chronic illnesses and diseases.

► Choose the Method for Category Classification

First, select the conditions you are going to sample. Then determine how to classify them. For example, if you look at fractures of the humerus, you might assign a code of 812, representing the major International Classification of Diseases, 9th revision (ICD-9), code that describes that condition. Because this is primarily an internal study, any classification format will suffice.

► Determine a Severity Level

Next, select a severity level. This is important because the more involved a specific treatment protocol or the greater the morbidity level, the more complex the treatment becomes and the more it is likely to cost. For example, a broken humerus can be a simple break or a compound fracture. It can occur in someone young and in good health or a diabetic in poor health. Each condition would prompt a different treatment protocol. It is suggested that five levels of severity, with 1 being the least severe and 5 being the most severe, be used.

► Select the Codes to Be Included

Next, decide what method you will use to determine which procedure codes to include in the study. You can do this by examining historical practice information and using those codes most commonly related to the

Using a sample methodology, determine what procedure codes have been reported when treating illnesses within this classification.

treatment protocol. National databases that contain the most common procedures recommended for use in specific treatment protocols are also available. The idea is to get the best overall representation possible. Most practices use historical data from within the practice. In most cases, you should only have to examine 10 charts for each classification/severity combination.

► Assign Individual Frequency

Count the number of times each procedure is reported for the sample set.

After you obtain a sampling of data for the specific condition/severity level, identify the individual procedures reported and assign frequencies to each. For example, when looking at the treatment for a hip replacement, it is necessary to include all procedures associated with the diagnoses and treatment, such as X-rays, surgeries, follow-up visits, supplies, and physical therapy. The most common method is to simply list each procedure reported in column 1 of a spreadsheet, add up the number of times that procedure is reported for each case, and put that frequency in column 2.

► Calculate Total and Average Costs

Finally, using the data from the cost accounting analysis, total the costs based on the frequency of the procedure and divide by the sample size to get the average cost per procedure.

Having already performed a procedural cost accounting analysis, you already know the actual line-item cost for each procedure the practice performs. So, in column 3, insert this cost value next to each procedure. Then, multiply the cost by the frequency and calculate the total cost for the sample. Next, divide the total cost by the number of records in the sample set to calculate the average cost per procedure. Finally, divide the total cost amount for each code into the number of records used in the sample. This will result in a value that equals the average cost per procedure performed for that classification.

CASE STUDY: HUMERUS FRACTURE

This case study exemplifies a typical treatment episode for a fracture of the humerus. The first steps are to assign an identifier, modify it for severity, and then determine the method for selecting the procedures.

In this case, you will use the primary ICD-9 code of 812 to classify this case. Then, because this represents a stable, nonsurgical fracture requiring closed reduction, you will give it a severity rating of 3, making the classification identifier 812-3. Finally, in order to develop a data set, you will pull the charts for the last seven patients who were treated for this particular diagnosis and severity.

Log the Procedures

Begin by building a spreadsheet that lists all of the codes reported for this classification.

Using a spreadsheet model, list all of the procedure codes (including modifiers) that were performed to treat this condition in column 1. This includes office visits, clinical procedures, diagnostic procedures, and services such as casting and injections. In column 2, insert a description for this procedure code. When you're done, your list may look something like that shown in Exhibit 5.1.

Determine Average Frequencies

Total up the number of times each procedure has been reported. For supply codes, simply total the cost amount. Then divide by the number of records in the sample to get the average frequency.

Next, if you are tabulating on paper, put a little hash mark next to the procedure code each time it has been performed. If you are using a spreadsheet, put the totals in the next column. The goal is to determine the total number of times the procedure has been performed. For the supply codes, such as 99070, list each supply in a separate column along with the estimated purchase cost for each item. For example, you want to figure in the cost of casting material and other such supplies not necessarily included in the cost of the procedure.

When done, divide the total frequency by 7. This results in the average frequency for each procedure and for each procedural occurrence for this diagnostic category.

Your table may now look Exhibit 5.2.

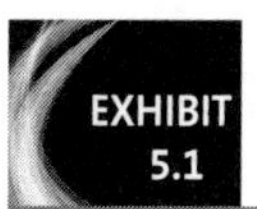

Procedure Codes Reported for Classification 812-3

Code	Description
99204	Office/outpatient visit, new
73060	X-ray exam of humerus
29065	Application of long arm cast
99213	Office/outpatient visit, established
29700	Removal/revision of cast
97039	Physical therapy treatment
99070	Supplies

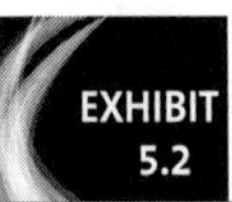

Cost Calculations for Classification 812-3

Code	Description	Total Freq	Average Freq
99204	Office/outpatient visit, new	5	.71
99203	Office/outpatient visit, new	2	.29
73060	X-ray exam of humerus	16	2.29
29065	Application of long arm cast	10	1.43
99213	Office/outpatient visit, established	28	4.00
29700	Removal/revision of cast	11	1.57
97039	Physical therapy treatment	28	4.00
99070	Supplies	$360.54	$51.51

Using the cost analysis, assign the line-item cost amount based upon the specific procedure code.

Assign Procedural Costs

Procedural costs are assigned during the cost accounting procedure, as outlined in the cost accounting section. Before proceeding, you must first conduct the cost accounting analysis in order to determine the cost per relative value unit and the cost per procedure. In column 4, put the line-item costs obtained from this cost accounting step (see Exhibit 5.3).

Multiply the average frequency by the unit cost to get the average cost per line item.

Calculate Total Cost

Multiply the unit cost by the frequency to obtain the total cost per procedure. Then take the sum of the products to calculate the total cost for this diagnostic category or treatment protocol (see Exhibit 5.4).

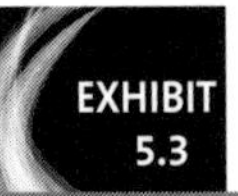

Assignment of Line-Item Cost per Procedure Code

Code	Description	Freq	Unit Cost
99204	Office/outpatient visit, new	.71	$45.50
99203	Office/outpatient visit, new	.29	$31.14
73060	X-ray exam of humerus	2.29	$11.01
29065	Application of long arm cast	1.43	$38.54
99213	Office/outpatient visit, established	4.00	$17.06
29700	Removal/revision of cast	1.57	$17.01
97039	Physical therapy treatment	4.00	$6.40
99070	Supplies		$51.51

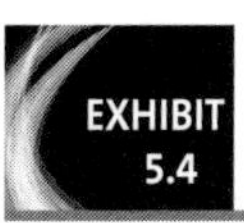

EXHIBIT 5.4 Calculation of Total Cost per Procedure Code

Code	Description	Freq	Unit Cost	Total Cost
99204	Office/outpatient visit, new	.71	$45.50	$32.31
99203	Office/outpatient visit, new	.29	$31.14	$9.03
73060	X-ray exam of humerus	2.29	$11.01	$25.21
29065	Application of long arm cast	1.43	$38.54	$55.11
99213	Office/outpatient visit, established	4.00	$17.06	$68.24
29700	Removal/revision of cast	1.57	$17.01	$26.71
97039	Physical therapy treatment	4.00	$6.40	$25.60
99070	Supplies		$51.51	$51.51
TOTAL				$293.72

You now know that there is a hard cost of $293.72 to treat a fractured humerus with a severity of 3. Now, what do you do with this information?

Global pricing is a new concept and, as such, presents the practice with an excellent opportunity for proactive planning.

PRACTICAL USES FOR GLOBAL PRICING

Although the original design for the global pricing model was to determine the feasibility for use under Medicare DRGs, the practical applications go far beyond the original objective. With an understanding of the methodology for applying the cost analysis, it will be much simpler to get to the global costing results than most practices may have considered. With a global costing model, your practice is in a position to apply the information to a variety of areas that deal not only with insurance and payer contracting but also with issues of quality assurance, cost control, and containment.

Bidding on Managed Care Contracts

Medicaid has already instituted global pricing concepts in some states where providers have found themselves in bidding wars with other providers. Knowledge of what it costs to treat a condition is critical to understanding the profitability of bidding for specific conditions and treatment protocols. In many cases, practices underbid to get a contract and then lose a great deal of money. The Oxford Group set several standards for this type of contracting that have proven very successful in

If you know the "drop dead" price at which profitability turns to financial loss, you can never lose on a global contract.

other public and private enterprises. This process was at the heart of the CMS demonstration project.

Medical practices are going to find themselves in the same position as other businesses when it comes to submitting competitive bids in order to provide services to end users. Patients, for the most part, do not pay their own healthcare bills. They are usually represented by large alliances, such as insurance companies. It is reasonable to believe that these alliances, acting in a business-like manner, are going to begin the process of competitive bidding on behalf of their subscribers.

Medical practices that are in a position to respond appropriately will have a better chance of financial survival, for two reasons. First, if they get the contract, they know they will be making a profit based on their calculated costs. Second, if they don't get the contract, they know they won't be losing money every time they treat someone within that particular diagnostic category.

Negotiating with Carriers

The key to successful negotiation is leverage and a defensible methodology.

A common complaint among smaller medical practices is that the managed care companies are not willing to negotiate contract terms and conditions. Although many managed care contracts appear to be nonnegotiable to these smaller practices, larger groups or physician organizations are in a position to negotiate more than they may realize. Most payers do not negotiate seriously with providers because the providers rarely have defensible methodologies to support their arguments. It is not enough to tell a managed care carrier that the fee is "too low" without being able to back up that statement. These types of analyses can produce acceptable methodologies that are understandable to both sides.

The resource-based relative value scale is nationally accepted as an industry standard.

Because you are using the resource-based relative value scale, the most widely accepted relative value scale, and because you are applying standard mathematical and accounting principles that can be duplicated, it is much easier to present a defensible case. Insurance companies do not have a viable business without subscribers, and subscribers will not stay with an insurance company if they are not able to see a physician with whom they are comfortable. Presenting standard, defensible, and acceptable models such as this has helped many medical providers negotiate acceptable contracts with managed care organizations and other similar payers.

Clinical Outcomes

As global pricing becomes a more common practice, national databases that contain average costs for treating specific diagnostic categories or conditions will appear. Knowing where the practice stands in comparison with the national average can provide the incentive to become more cost effective and more efficient and to have a baseline of information for bidding strategies.

From the standpoint of quality assurance, you can ensure that your treatment protocols provide your patients with the best possible outcomes.

This is most effective for clinical outcome data and research. Comparing the treatment protocol for a diagnostic category or condition with that of other local physicians can help to develop treatment guidelines that will ensure the best quality of care for patients.

Clinical Reengineering

A very important outcome of this type of analysis is the ability to more closely scrutinize the way the practice uses resources. Medical practices use clinical engineering to "tighten up" their clinical procedures and to become more efficient without compromising patient care or treatment outcomes.

Clinical reengineering is a very important area of cost control that is often overlooked in the medical practice.

In the following example, a practice decided to closely examine its treatment protocol, comparing what they did to what was done by other orthopedic specialists. What follows demonstrates how this process can become valuable within the practice. Let's compare Exhibit 5.5 with Exhibit 5.4 and see what changes the practice made to lower its cost in treating this condition.

1. **Reduce the number of 99213 visits.** Here, the practice converted two 99213 visits to 99212 visits and one to a 99211 visit. This was not only more cost effective for the practice but also reduced waiting time for the patient, particularly in the case of the 99211, where it was not necessary for the physician to be present. A physician's assistant, nurse practitioner, or the office registered nurse could handle this final exam. While this was happening, the physician was seeing another patient, generating revenue for that visit and thereby reducing the opportunity cost associated with this final visit.

2. **Reduce the number of physical therapy visits from four to one.** Through consultation with a national database, the staff found that it was as effective to train the patient how to do his or her

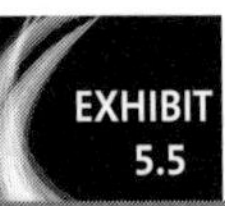

EXHIBIT 5.5 Example of Clinical Reengineering

Code	Description	Freq	Unit Cost	Total Cost
99204	Office/outpatient visit, new	.71	$45.50	$32.31
99203	Office/outpatient visit, new	.29	$31.14	$9.03
73060	X-ray exam of humerus	2.29	$11.01	$25.21
29065	Application of long arm cast	1.43	$38.54	$55.11
99213	*Office/outpatient visit, established*	*1.00*	*$17.06*	*$17.06*
99212	*Office/outpatient visit, established*	*2.00*	*$12.37*	*$24.74*
99211	*Office/outpatient visit, established*	*1.00*	*$6.68*	*$6.68*
29700	Removal/revision of cast	1.57	$17.01	$26.71
97039	*Physical therapy treatment*	*1.00*	*$6.40*	*$6.40*
99070	*Supplies*			*$22.15*
TOTAL				$225.50

Note: Italic type indicates line items for which a reduction in services would likely be appropriate.

own therapy for this condition on the first visit. Then they sent the patient home with a dumbbell to continue strength and range-of-motion training on his or her own. After several treatments and after tracking several cases, the outcomes for patients receiving one physical therapy and training session was as good as for those receiving four of the same sessions.

3. **Reduce the amount spent on additional or supportive supplies.** The practice replaced more expensive products with generic ones and chose reusable, as opposed to disposable, products in certain circumstances, reducing the amount of supplies used.

This reengineering process saved the practice $68.32 for this condition. Such steps make it possible for the practice to be more competitive while bidding, increase the practice's profits under global contracts, or both.

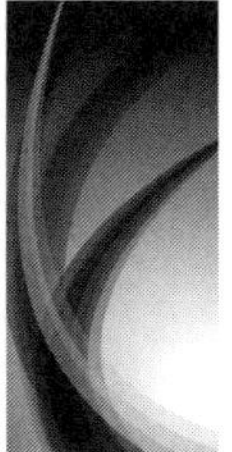

CHAPTER 6

Measuring Physician Productivity

Like it or not, productivity is a measure of the final financial contribution the provider makes to the practice. It's about what is left after the dust settles and both revenue and expenses have been considered. However, productivity is not a measure of how hard one works, how much revenue one generates, or how sick one's patients are. Most importantly, productivity is not a measure of the human value of a physician. That can only be measured by compassion and commitment.

In the past, when the issue of physician productivity was discussed, people heard "physician compensation." For many years, physician compensation was based almost exclusively on generated revenue and seniority and specifically not based upon productivity. For example, if one physician generated 30 percent of the revenue, she or he was entitled to 30 percent of the compensation and bonus distribution. This method left much to be desired with respect to the utilization of resources within a practice. In other words, there was no consideration for expenses. For example, using a standard linear distribution model, in a five-physician practice, one would expect to see each physician generating exactly 20 percent of the revenue for the practice. In this case, each physician would receive an equal share of the compensation and bonuses. The problem occurs when a physician consumes more resources than the revenue generated. This consumption of resources translates to costs, or the portion of the practice's expenses that can be directly attributed to that physician.

By using known data, such as the relative value unit amounts and the annual frequency for the procedures performed by the physician, you can calculate ratios that accurately measure true productivity.

Using relative value scale (RVS) analysis, specifically the resource-based relative value scale (RBRVS) data set, one can effectively measure the amount of work effort expended and the amount of resources consumed by each physician. By determining how frequently each physician performs a procedure, you can use RVS analysis techniques to calculate the total number of relative value units (RVUs) each physician reports. Because each RVU is a measure of resource consumption, or cost, you can develop a pattern of expense as well as generated revenue for each physician in the practice. Then, by building a ratio of revenue to cost, you can accurately measure the physician's productivity and real contribution to the practice's bottom line.

The best use of a productivity analysis is to help less productive physicians become more productive.

In reviewing this methodology, you are only looking at and applying cost/revenue data. No consideration is made for specialty, administrative duties, alternate revenue sources, or the like. Therefore, it may not be prudent to use only these calculations to determine the compensation and bonus distribution for the physician. In fact, building compensation models is not the best use of the productivity calculations. Increasing productivity for individual providers results in an increase in the overall productivity of the practice. Therefore, by studying the most productive physicians and applying his or her techniques to those who are less productive, overall productivity for the practice will increase and everyone involved will benefit.

WHAT IS PRODUCTIVITY?

Productivity is a measurement of the relationship between what comes in (revenue) and what goes out (expenses).

Productivity, in most industries, is measured by comparing income to expense. In manufacturing, for example, productivity is measured by the cost per output in relation to the fee charged for the item. Excluding quality issues for the moment, this allows the manufacturing facility to identify the efficiency of its processes. In healthcare, particularly the physician's office, productivity is reviewed using a relative measurement of cost based upon a relative value scale. In this sense, you are depending upon an outside study to generalize the work-related efforts and cost to deliver an individual service or perform a specific procedure, that is, the practice's product. In the best practices, this concept is applied to cost accounting techniques in order to determine the reasonability of the fees that are charged.

In measuring productivity, you are looking at what you generate in revenues (which is tied in some degree to costs) and what it costs to deliver the service that generates that fee. In considering the compensation of a medical practice's owners and/or the generators of the revenue, that is,

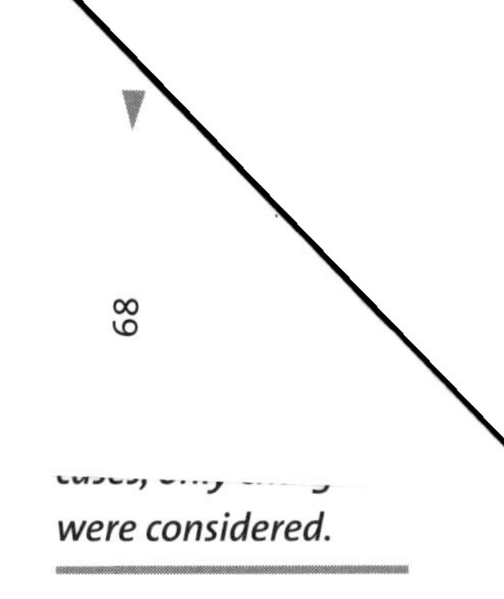

the providers, you also look at profitability. This is also tied into the cost revenue ratio.

were considered.

► Old School

Many years ago, productivity was determined based solely on generation of revenue, without consideration for the cost of generating that revenue. Until the advent of the RBRVS, this was the only option open to many practices. Hence, compensation was also based upon this method. Although revenue is certainly important for the sustenance of the practice, the value of the service or product is not fairly measured without considering all sides of the equation, including (and, critically, in healthcare) the quality of the product. In some cases, charges rather than revenue were used, and this only created a much greater margin of error because charges, in many cases, have little to do with revenue.

► New School

With the introduction and further refining of the RBRVS, it is easier, more accessible, and more affordable for practices to look at productivity using this particular model of global expense and cost measurement. With respect to building a relational model, finances in the medical practice can be measured in three general ways:

- Gross charges;
- Gross collections (gross revenues); or
- Gross profit.

Expenses can also be measured in three general ways:

- Tracked contribution;
- Time–motion studies; or
- RBRVS databases.

Gross charges are easy to measure, unless the practice bills using multiple fee schedules. Although gross charges prevent physicians from being punished by a poor billing and collection process, it is moot if the practice establishes its fee schedule using the resource-based relative value scale.

MEASURING PRODUCTION

Gross charges are commonly used in developing physician productivity studies because they provide for a common denominator or a consistent component for the left side of the equation. Gross charges are obtained by multiplying the commercial fee schedule by the number of times the procedure is performed and then calculating the sum of the products. However, this can be difficult if the practice bills using multiple fee schedules for different providers. Using gross charges takes the burden of the billing and collection process (and, many times, the penalty for a poor system) away from the physicians. It also puts more of a burden on the value of the fee schedule itself. In fact, it can be argued that using the gross charges simply measures the discrepancy within the fee schedule. For example, a physician within a group who delivers specific services where the fees are not relative to the fees of the other physicians can have an impact on the productivity analysis. Another negative is that if the fee schedule is developed using the RBRVS or based upon a factor of the Medicare fee schedule amount, each provider will have exactly the same level of productivity. Using this measurement can also mask problems that may occur with coding and billing issues related to specific providers. For example, if one provider is being regularly denied based upon poor documentation, coding errors, or payer anomalies, the use of gross charges will prevent this from being discovered and will unfairly credit that provider for services that are not being paid.

Gross revenue, or collections, is very effective for calculating profit/loss by physician. It is, however, subject to accounts receivable problems and inordinate collection efforts that fall outside the reporting period.

Gross revenue, or gross collections, is also commonly used to develop physician productivity studies because many practices have the ability to track procedural revenue by physician. Use of this measurement allows for profit/loss measurement by physician. If gross revenue is to be used, it is recommended that it be done in a manner that assigns actual tracked revenue data for each physician. This method takes into account the efficiency of the billing and collections process and the staff efforts involved. Unfortunately, it holds the physician accountable for what is often a poor system for billing and collections, especially in practice management companies and hospital-owned physician practices, where poorly managed systems and cost shifting unfairly add expense to the physician practice component. Although this appears to be a straightforward method for calculating revenue, some practices experience problems related to accounts receivable (A/R) days and collection efforts that fall outside the collection period. For example, the practice may report A/R days of 62, meaning that it takes approximately 62 days after the billing submission to collect the payment. If, for example, the period that measures frequency runs from January 1 through December 31, the collections will be recorded only for those frequencies from March 1 through December 31. The other issue deals with out-of-period collection efforts. This might occur when the practice begins collecting payments on claims that are aged prior to the period that represents the performance and billing period.

Gross profit looks at what is left after all of the expenses, including write-offs, disallowances, fixed and variable expenses, depreciation, and taxes, have been subtracted. Although this combines some of the problems found in the prior two methods, it can be important when considering compensation. The problem with this method is standardization because there are many ways to calculate gross profit.

Gross profit is the most variable of the three models and is very difficult to standardize.

MEASURING EXPENSES

Activity-based costing (ABC), also referred to as "tracked contribution," requires a sophisticated accounting and/or practice management system that tracks costs as direct expenses by physician. More often than not, this involves the use of outside consultants to both establish and monitor the study. This includes distribution of square feet of office space, time utilization of assigned staff, and shared distribution of common expense categories. Some teaching facilities attempt to isolate costs in this fashion, as do some specialized groups. For the most part, however, the typical medical practice is not capable of this level of differentiation. This method requires the ability to assess specific lengths of time for procedures and to allocate direct expenses based upon the time contributed by each resource component. Some studies are available that attempt to assign cost based on ABC; however, the greatest difficulty comes in the effort to identify, or define, the "typical" medical practice and how to adjust the studies based on an "atypical" finding.

Tracked contribution requires a fairly sophisticated accounting system.

Time–motion studies, also referred to as efficiency-flow analyses, use automated and portable computer tracking hardware to measure all aspects of a practice's operational components. Time–motion studies, although normally very accurate, are also very expensive, very complicated, and can vary in design and report methodology. Although effective for flow-charting specific processes in specific time increments, this type of study is not effective when looking at the entire practice as a dynamic business process.

Time–motion studies may very well be the most accurate of all methods. This type of study is also the most expensive, intrusive, and variable of reporting methodologies.

The *RBRVS,* although controversial with respect to its design methodology, has been standardized within the industry and has undergone extensive refinement in its first 10 years. There is much controversy over the accuracy of the RVU components (particularly the work component). However, as long as RBRVS is used vertically (within the same entity) and not extrapolated horizontally (as in between different entities), it can be very accurate and effective. The database is in the public domain, is readily available, and, after a general study of the development method, is relatively easy and inexpensive to use. Because it is a relational model based upon resources instead of costs (at least that is the design), it is very effective when moving dynamics are measured within the same data universe, or medical practice. Although the RBRVS-based analysis looks at a static slice of time, it is applicable across a more global dynamic business model.

MEASURING PRODUCTIVITY

As long as the data are available, you can measure productivity by individual provider.

Using the above information, you can effectively measure the clinical productivity of any individual provider of medical services, as long as the information for that provider is tracked properly. A key word here is *clinical* because the RBRVS is a clinical-based study. Therefore, nonclinical revenues and expenses, such as those involving research or administration, are not considered.

Productivity is measured by first evaluating the relationship between generated revenue and consumed resources, or expenses. If your practice tracks frequencies by provider, you can develop a revenue side and an RVU-based cost side for each. By identifying a control group (against which the provider will be measured), you can look at individual contribution to revenue and cost as a relationship to that group. This can be the entire practice entity, a multiple-practice organization, a department, or even a provider if activity-based accounting is available. Then, by building a relationship between those two ratios, you can develop a true relationship of revenue to cost as it applies to that specific universe. Because you are measuring clinical components using ratios in a closed system, full-time equivalent (FTE) factors are not considered. As presented here, productivity (as a ratio), rather than just measuring absolute revenue or absolute expense, quantifies the relationship for each provider in relation to the entire group. Although this should not be used for the final compensation model by itself, it does provide a defensible benchmark for initiating the process and measuring individual productivity.

If cost per provider can be calculated, then measuring profitability is a logical and simple step.

Profitability, although not as effective in measuring pure productivity, is an effective way to measure relative productivity for the purpose of compensation/bonus plans. This method is applicable providing it also employs an RBRVS-based cost analysis. In this model, global expense data and specific provider data are used in order to develop a cost-per-RVU value. This value is applied to line-item services and procedures by multiplying the cost for that procedure by its individual RVU value. Again, because this is based upon the RBRVS and clinical contribution, it eliminates the need for FTE consideration.

PHYSICIAN PRODUCTION MODELS

To determine production for each physician, you will need:

- Total generated charge and revenue
- Total RVU utilization for total RVUs, work RVUs, and practice expense RVUs

If you have access to the information, you can measure productivity by defining the control (or target) group.

For each control location or group, you will need the same information. A control group or location is the data set against which the selected group is compared. For example, if you have four physicians working at one location, you may use the location as the control group. In this case, you can measure the performance of each physician against the group of physicians at that location. If there are many locations, you can measure the performance of the physicians in a specific location against all locations. In any case, the amount of data required will depend upon these two factors.

In calculating RVU amounts, remember that it is critical to factor in the RVU value for any associated modifiers. For example, if a physician regularly bills for surgical assists using modifier 81 and the RVUs are not being adjusted appropriately (however that might occur), that provider will be held responsible for the full RVU value (consumption) yet only credited for approximately 15 percent to 25 percent of the revenue, potentially significantly understating his or her productivity.

Don't forget the importance of adjusting the relative value unit value for the modifier factor.

In the following example, data from four physicians working in the same practice are used. It is assumed that all physicians work full time and, although they share the same specialty, each physician also performs different procedures exclusive from the others and also shares common procedures. Charges are calculated by summing the products of the fees and multiplying this by the frequencies; revenue is provided by the practice. The following four tables represent a sampling of codes for each physician for a period of the most recent year.

Sample Study – Physician 1

Code	Fee	TPY	Work RVU	PE RVU	MP RVU	Sum RVU	Total RVUs	Total Work RVU	Total Charge
10060	$75	159	1.12	0.44	0.04	1.60	254.40	178.08	$11,925
10061	$175	10	2.48	0.64	0.06	3.18	31.80	24.80	$1,750
10120	$75	27	1.19	0.46	0.05	1.70	45.90	32.13	$2,025
10121	$185	97	2.64	1.00	0.12	3.76	364.72	256.08	$17,945
10140	$55	133	1.48	0.48	0.05	2.01	267.33	196.84	$7,315
10160	$55	62	1.15	0.38	0.05	1.58	97.96	71.30	$3,410
11000	$55	72	0.91	0.40	0.04	1.35	97.20	65.52	$3,960
11040	$65	16	0.50	0.40	0.04	0.94	15.04	8.00	$1,040
11042	$135	179	1.12	0.65	0.08	1.85	331.15	200.48	$24,165
TOTALS							1505.50	1033.23	$73,535

- Total charges = $73,535
- Total revenue = $50,371
- Total RVU = 1,505.50
- Total work RVU = 1033.23
- Ratio of work RVU to total RVU = 68.6 percent

Sample Study – Physician 2

Code	Fee	TPY	Work RVU	PE RVU	MP RVU	Sum RVU	Total RVUs	Total Work RVU	Total Charge
11050	$35	400	0.43	0.37	0.03	0.83	332.00	172.00	$14,000
11051	$45	212	0.66	0.50	0.05	1.21	256.52	139.92	$9,540
11052	$52	111	0.86	0.41	0.04	1.31	145.41	95.46	$5,772
11420	$150	41	1.01	0.52	0.05	1.58	64.78	41.41	$6,150
11421	$200	92	1.48	0.71	0.07	2.26	207.92	136.16	$18,400
11422	$250	66	1.71	0.94	0.10	2.75	181.50	112.86	$16,500
11423	$300	35	2.12	1.31	0.15	3.58	125.30	74.20	$10,500
11424	$350	3	2.57	1.39	0.16	4.12	12.36	7.71	$1,050
11602	$160	1	2.04	1.82	0.16	4.02	4.02	2.04	$160
11606	$400	1	3.38	3.11	0.49	6.98	6.98	3.38	$400
TOTALS							1336.79	785.14	$82,472

- Total charges = $82,472
- Total revenue = $58,555
- Total RVU = 1,336.79
- Total work RVU = 785.14
- Ratio of work RVU to total RVU = 58.7 percent

Sample Study – Physician 3

Code	Fee	TPY	Work RVU	PE RVU	MP RVU	Sum RVU	Total RVUs	Total Work RVUs	Total Charge
11620	$210	21	1.29	1.34	0.12	2.75	57.75	27.09	$4,410
11621	$260	27	1.92	1.75	0.16	3.83	103.41	51.84	$7,020
11622	$310	19	2.29	2.20	0.19	4.68	88.92	43.51	$5,890
11623	$360	28	2.88	2.58	0.25	5.71	159.88	80.64	$10,080
11624	$410	26	3.38	3.21	0.32	6.91	179.66	87.88	$10,660
11700	$26	107	0.32	0.32	0.03	0.67	71.69	34.24	$2,782
11701	$15	111	0.23	0.23	0.02	0.48	53.28	25.53	$1,665
11710	$35	161	0.32	0.32	0.03	0.67	107.87	51.52	$5,635
11711	$15	371	0.20	0.19	0.02	0.41	152.11	74.20	$5,565
11730	$95	158	1.13	0.45	0.04	1.62	255.96	178.54	$15,010
TOTALS							1230.53	654.99	$68,717

- Total charges = $68,717
- Total revenue = $46,177
- Total RVU = 1,230.53
- Total work RVU = 654.99
- Ratio of work RVU to total RVU = 53.2 percent

Sample Study – Physician 4

Code	Fee	TPY	Work RVU	PE RVU	MP RVU	Sum RVU	Total RVUs	Total Work RVUs	Total Charge
11920	$195	21	1.61	1.18	0.23	3.02	63.42	33.81	$4,095
17000	$75	117	0.64	0.42	0.03	1.09	127.53	74.88	$8,775
17001	$50	67	0.19	0.19	0.02	0.40	26.80	12.73	$3,350
20550	$37	142	0.86	0.38	0.04	1.28	181.76	122.12	$5,254
20600	$37	136	0.66	0.47	0.05	1.18	160.48	89.76	$5,032
20605	$45	301	0.68	0.45	0.05	1.18	355.18	204.68	$13,545
20650	$45	317	2.07	1.08	0.14	3.29	1042.93	656.19	$14,265
20670	$195	22	1.69	0.74	0.11	2.54	55.88	37.18	$4,290
20680	$485	16	3.25	3.33	0.51	7.09	113.44	52.00	$7,760
28010	$125	11	2.97	3.62	0.33	6.92	76.12	32.67	$1,375
TOTALS							2203.54	1316.02	$67,741

- Total charges = $67,741
- Total revenue = $34,548
- Total RVU = 2,203.54
- Total work RVU = 1,316.02
- Ratio of work RVU to total RVU = 59.7 percent

CALCULATING COLLECTION PERCENT BY PROVIDER

When calculating the collection percent by provider, the first step is to identify the difference between gross charges and revenue (collections) per provider (Exhibit 6.1). This says volumes about the processes that include coding, billing, and collections. Gross charges are used because they provide a somewhat stable fulcrum for this type of calculation.

Exhibit 6.1 indicates a range of collection percentages from a low of 51 percent to a high of 70.15 percent. In a practice where there is a similarity in specialties and homogeneity with regard to patient characteristics and payer mix, this type of variance is indicative of coding problems. In this example, based on volume of services, Doc 4 is responsible for degrading the collection amount for the entire practice.

IDENTIFYING RESOURCE CONSUMPTION

Resource consumption is defined by RBRVS. Therefore, the total calculated RVUs by provider are entered. Then, the total amount for each column, which in this example is the control group, is calculated. For this example, assume that you have access to actual revenue generated for each physician (Exhibit 6.2).

Distribute Data by Control Totals

The next step is to develop distribution relationships by dividing each provider's values by the control group totals. In this case, the control group is represented by the totals for the group (Exhibit 6.3).

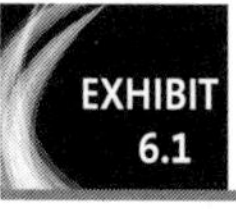

Collection Ratio by Provider

Physician	Gross Charges	Generated Revenue	Collection	Variance from Practice
Doc 1	$73,535	$50,371	68.50%	106.00%
Doc 2	$83,472	$58,555	70.15%	108.55%
Doc 3	$68,717	$46,177	67.20%	103.98%
Doc 4	$67,741	$34,548	51.00%	78.92%
TOTALS	$293,465	$189,651	64.62%	

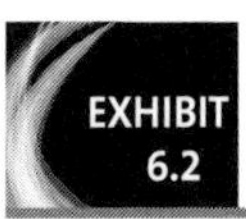
EXHIBIT 6.2

Revenue and Utilization by Doc

Physician	Gross Charges	Generated Revenue	Resource Expenditure
Doc 1	$73,535	$50,371	1505.50
Doc 2	$83,472	$58,555	1336.79
Doc 3	$68,717	$46,177	1230.53
Doc 4	$67,741	$34,548	2203.54
TOTALS	$293,465	$189,651	6276.36

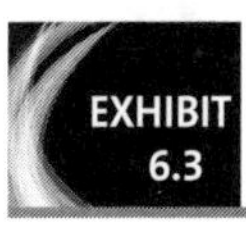
EXHIBIT 6.3

Distribution of Revenues and Resources by Doc

Physician	Generated Revenue	Resource Expenditure	Revenue of Total	Resource of Total
Doc 1	$50,371	1505.50	26.56%	23.99%
Doc 2	$58,555	1336.79	30.88%	21.30%
Doc 3	$46,177	1230.53	24.35%	19.61%
Doc 4	$34,548	2203.54	18.22%	35.11%
TOTALS	$189,651	6276.36	100.00%	100.00%

► Build Revenue-to-Utilization Ratios

The ratio of revenue as a percent of the total to RVUs as a percent of the total is used to define productivity (Exhibit 6.4). There are two ways to measure this marker: absolute and relative. Absolute productivity defines the relationship without consideration for productivity within the control group or, in this case, the practice. Relative productivity measures the relationship of the individual physician's productivity to that of the practice.

By developing a productivity ratio, you can quickly identify those physicians whose consumption of resources exceeds their generation of revenue as a percent of the group totals.

This ratio allows you to determine the relative productivity of the physician compared with the mean productivity of the control group. If the ratio is greater than 1, the physician is generally considered productive. If the ratio is less than 1, the physician is considered less productive. To determine the provider's productivity as it relates to other members of the group, first divide the total ratio by the number of records (4.2319/4 = 1.06) and compare individual ratios to that value. If the

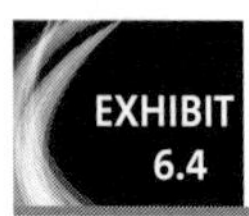
EXHIBIT 6.4

Building the Revenue-to-Resource Ratio

Physician	Generated Revenue	Resource Expenditure	Revenue of Total	Resource of Total	Absolute Productivity	Relative Productivity
Doc 1	$50,371	1505.50	25.06%	23.99%	1.04	0.99
Doc 2	$58,555	1336.79	28.44%	21.30%	1.34	1.26
Doc 3	$46,177	1230.53	23.42%	19.61%	1.19	1.13
Doc 4	$34,548	2203.54	23.08%	35.11%	0.66	0.62
TOTALS	$189,651	6276.36	100.00%	100.00%	4.23	

ratio is greater than the mean, the provider is generally more productive than average for the group. A ratio that is less than this value indicates a productivity level that is less than average for the group. In this example, only Doc 4 is below the absolute mean productivity level and both Doc 1 and Doc 4 are less productive than average for the group. An important point to note here is that negative productivity does not always translate into negative profitability.

PHYSICIAN COMPENSATION CONSIDERATIONS

Productivity ratios, as developed here, provide the foundation for compensation models. Under most circumstances, however, you will also need to factor in other considerations to ensure equity among providers.

It is important to remember that revenue-to-utilization ratios measure productivity relative to the control group and do not measure profitability of the individual providers. The productivity ratio is an important benchmark when you begin the compensation process. Unless an argument is made as to the validity of either the RBRVS or the method for determining revenue, this type of model is highly defensible. Again, however, it is important to remember that this model is not a stand-alone end-all for compensation calculations because it represents a *clinical* productivity model only. Administrative duties, ownership, seniority, and other issues must be taken into consideration when developing a full compensation package for a provider.

Calculate Distribution Amounts

Finally, take the ratio distribution line item for each physician and divide it by the total in the last row (Exhibit 6.5). This will redistribute the ratios to build a normal distribution amount for each physician.

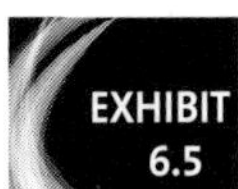

EXHIBIT 6.5

Calculating Distribution from Productivity Ratio

Physician	Generated Revenue	Resource Expenditure	Revenue of Total	Resource of Total	Ratio	Distribution
Doc 1	$50,371	1505.50	26.56%	23.99%	1.107	25.65%
Doc 2	$58,555	1336.79	30.88%	21.30%	1.450	33.57%
Doc 3	$46,177	1230.53	24.35%	19.61%	1.242	28.76%
Doc 4	$34,548	2203.54	18.22%	35.11%	0.519	12.02%
TOTALS	$189,651	6276.36	100.00%	100.00%	4.318	100.00%

In this example, if you were to base compensation solely on generated revenue, the variance between the highest and the lowest would be a factor of approximately 12.5 percent. When you examine the relative resource utilization for each provider, or their expense contribution, there is a significant variance from the relationship of generated revenue. In this example, if you use only RVUs, Doc 4 would get a significantly higher, yet disproportionate, share of the pool. Yet, when you factor this with revenue, the results are considerably different. This could be due to payer mix, specialty, or even coding problems that result in denials and rejections for services provided. In any case, as productivity is defined here, Doc 4 is the least productive of the group and, unless there are other overriding reasons, may be considered for a lower compensation value. Using productivity, the variance between the lowest and highest values climbs to approximately 21 percent, yet this indicates a more balanced methodology for considering overall contribution to the group. It is important to note that you have not yet examined profitability; failing to do so means the possibility of including a provider who had a negative contribution to the bonus distribution pool.

Looking at the relationship between revenue and resources, you can see why the use of only revenue or only relative value units as a guide for compensation can be unfair to some within the group.

Using Profit/Loss to Calculate Productivity

It may be possible to measure profit/loss alone in order to calculate productivity providing you are measuring clinical-based services only. Additionally, actual revenues (or collections) tracked for each physician should be used so that the measure of profitability or loss is actual and not projected. All services, including ancillary services, should be tracked. Whether or not these services are used to calculate physician

When calculating profitability, it is important to include the revenue for all services, including ancillary services, which may be tracked separately.

compensation, the revenue they generate should also be applied to each physician's calculation because the resources to deliver those services have been calculated using the RVU values assigned to them. This would include the technical component–modified procedures because, although they result in charges, costs, and revenue, work RVUs are not assigned and therefore could skew productivity and the resulting profitability calculations.

If profitability is going to be considered for compensation, then collections must be tracked accurately.

Accurate tracking of collections is as important as accurate calculation of costs. Collections in particular can present certain challenges that must be overcome before this model can be applied to compensation. Actual revenue can be affected by collection techniques, coding and/or billing problems, A/R days, and managed care organization agreements. For example, some physicians may see certain populations whose insurance payments are not as favorable, and therefore actual collections may be less for those physicians than others within the group. This is particularly true for providers who focus on Medicare, Medicaid, or patients with coverage from a health maintenance organization (HMO).

Multiply the cost per relative value unit by the total relative value units for that provider to determine the provider's calculated expenses.

Calculate Cost per Provider

To calculate the total cost for an individual provider, take the total number of RVUs assigned to that provider and multiply it by the cost per RVU for the practice (Exhibit 6.6). This value was calculated during the cost analysis process. For this example, 36.6137 was used as the cost per RVU.

In some situations, this represents an oversimplification of the costing process. Many times, there are direct-expense considerations when calculating costs for providers. For example, in a multispecialty practice,

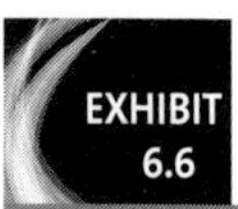

Calculating Cost per Provider

Physician	Generated Revenue	Resource Expenditure	Cost
Doc 1	$50,371	1505.50	**$55,122**
Doc 2	$58,555	1336.79	**$48,945**
Doc 3	$46,177	1230.53	**$45,054**
Doc 4	$34,548	2203.54	**$80,680**
TOTALS	$189,651	6276.36	**$229,801**

malpractice premiums may be assigned as a direct expense to each provider. In some cases, providers have certain medical staff that work only for them. For problems such as excess capacity, the calculated excess expense amount is divided equally among the providers. Much of this is discussed later in this chapter.

Calculate Profit or Loss

To calculate profit/loss, simply subtract the calculated cost from the tracked revenue.

In calculating the profit or loss for each physician as it relates to his or her productivity, subtract the cost amount from the revenue amount (Exhibit 6.7). In the case of charges, this most likely will not reflect a real value. If based upon actual collections, it more than likely will represent the actual realized profitability for each provider. Remember that this pertains only to clinical procedures and services that are included within the cost accounting table.

It can be tricky dealing with providers that post a loss. Because you normally don't charge providers to practice, you need to find a way to normalize the database. In most cases, deleting the record is the best way.

Exhibit 6.7 indicates that both Doc 1 and Doc 4 have posted a loss. This is not unusual for new physicians or nonphysician providers. In the case of an established physician, however, this can pose certain challenges to the practice. In calculating the profit/loss distribution, one of two options will normalize the database. The first is to delete the record for those providers who post a loss. This will distribute the positive balance (if there is one) to the remaining providers. This is the best option when more than one provider is posting a loss. The other option is simply to add the negative amount to each provider's total profit/loss value. This will zero out the profit/loss for the negative provider and redistribute the normalized values to the other providers. This is only recommended when only one provider is showing a loss.

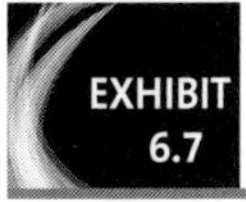

Calculating Profit/Loss by Provider

Physician	Generated Revenue	Resource Expenditure	Cost	P/L	Distrib
Doc 1	$50,371	1505.50	$55,122	–4,751	11.83%
Doc 2	$58,555	1336.79	$48,945	9,610	–23.94%
Doc 3	$46,177	1230.53	$45,054	1,123	–2.80%
Doc 4	$34,548	2203.54	$80,680	–46,132	114.90%
TOTALS	$189,651	6276.36	$229,801	–40,150	100.00%

By deleting the provider that posted a loss from the table, you can calculate a distribution amount for the remaining providers.

CALCULATE PROFIT DISTRIBUTION

Doc 1 and Doc 4 have been deleted from the table because they posted losses. Deleting them from the table ensures that they won't share in the bonus distribution for the practice and redistributes the remaining amount to the other providers. In this example, because the practice reported an overall loss, there is no profit sharing among the providers. If there were a surplus, however, it would be divided based upon the percent of profitability shown in the corresponding column in Exhibit 6.8.

PRACTICE EXAMPLE

Exhibit 6.9 is an example of a medical group consisting of 15 distinct medical providers.

Column 1 identifies the provider identification.

Column 2 identifies the revenue generated by that physician.

Column 3 represents the total RVUs assigned to each physician as a result of multiplying the individual RVU value for each procedure performed by the annual frequency attributed to that physician.

Column 4 contains the cost assigned to each physician. This value was obtained by multiplying the cost per RVU (42.21) times the total RVUs assigned to that physician.

Column 5 contains the profit/loss assigned to that physician. This value was obtained by subtracting the cost from the collected amount.

Column 6 contains the revenue-to-cost ratio. This value was obtained by dividing each physician's revenue by his or her assigned cost. These are absolute values and they are not relational, meaning that they represent only that specific physician's personal productivity without consideration for the other providers within the entity.

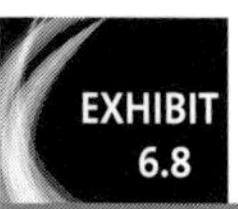

Calculating Profit Distribution by Provider

Physician	Generated Revenue	Resource Expenditure	Cost	P/L	Percent Distrib
Doc 2	\$58,555	1336.79	\$48,945	9,610	89.54%
Doc 3	\$46,177	1230.53	\$45,054	1,123	10.46%
TOTALS	\$104,732	2567.32	\$93,999	10,733	100.00%

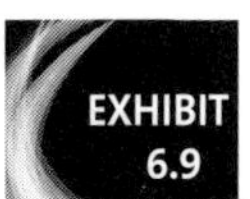

EXHIBIT 6.9 Productivity Table

ID	Gross Revenue	RVU	Cost	P/L	R/C Ratio	P/L Dist	Rev	RVU	Prod Ratio	Dist
1	$701,783	10,719	$452,449	249,334	1.551	16.45%	8.19%	6.41%	1.28	8.12%
2	$540,859	15,440	$651,722	−110,863	0.830	−7.32%	6.31%	9.24%	0.68	4.35%
3	$360,812	6,033	$254,653	106,159	1.417	7.01%	4.21%	3.61%	1.17	7.42%
4	$622,251	11,393	$480,899	141,352	1.294	9.33%	7.26%	6.82%	1.07	6.78%
5	$243,368	4,832	$203,959	39,409	1.193	2.60%	2.84%	2.89%	0.98	6.25%
6	$232,745	5,832	$246,169	−13,424	0.945	−0.89%	2.72%	3.49%	0.78	4.95%
7	$190,009	3,542	$149,508	40,501	1.271	2.67%	2.22%	2.12%	1.05	6.65%
8	$754,164	8,722	$368,156	386,008	2.048	25.47%	8.80%	5.22%	1.69	10.73%
9	$943,501	15,024	$634,163	309,338	1.488	20.41%	11.01%	8.99%	1.22	7.79%
10	$537,436	9,866	$416,444	120,992	1.291	7.98%	6.27%	5.90%	1.06	6.76%
11	$423,702	8,912	$376,176	47,526	1.126	3.14%	4.94%	5.33%	0.93	5.90%
12	$1,711,370	41,223	$1,740,023	−28,653	0.984	−1.89%	19.97%	24.67%	0.81	5.15%
13	$354,258	6,674	$281,710	72,548	1.258	4.79%	4.13%	3.99%	1.04	6.58%
14	$299,692	5,828	$246,000	53,692	1.218	3.54%	3.50%	3.49%	1.00	6.38%
15	$653,399	13,074	$551,854	101,545	1.184	6.70%	7.62%	7.82%	0.97	6.20%

Column 7 represents the distribution of the profit/loss across all physicians. This allows for a relative look at the contribution of each physician compared to the entire entity measured.

Column 8 represents that physician's revenue as a percent of the control group total.

Column 9 represents that physician's RVU utilization as a percent of the control group total.

Column 10 represents the ratio of the revenue percent to the RVU percent. This calculation more accurately represents actual productivity than does the calculation in column 6. Here, values below 1 represent a negative productivity compared to the mean productivity for the entire control group. Unlike the ratios in column 6, there are no absolute negative values because, irrespective of the provider's profitability, there is still a work effort and a charge value involved, even if no collections were realized.

Column 11 represents the theoretical bonus/compensation distribution percent. The value was obtained by dividing each revenue-to-RVU ratio by the sum of the products for that column. Again, using a normal distribution table, each physician would be entitled to 6.67 percent of the distribution amount. Note that the distribution values here are the same as those in column 7, although the ratios are different. The reason for this is that by using the RBRVS, the expenses are tied to costs through the assignment of RVUs, thus equating costs to RVUs and RVU calculations to expense calculations.

Revenue vs. Utilization

The data in series 1 in Exhibit 6.10 identify the revenue generated by each physician as a percent of the revenue generated for the control group. The data in series 2 indicate the RVUs consumed by each physician as a percent of the total RVUs consumed by the control group.

Exhibit 6.11 shows the percentages from Exhibit 6.10 as a ratio relative to each other, as calculated in Exhibit 6.9. Note that what appears to

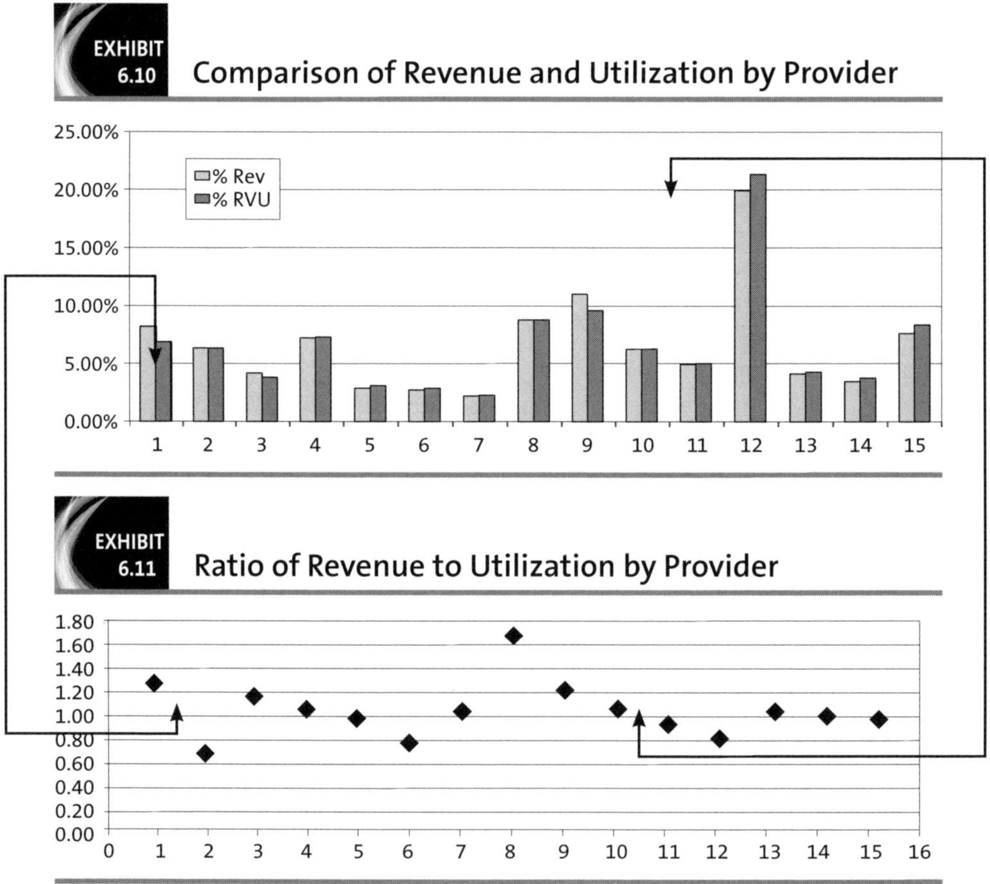

be a high level of productivity (Exhibit 6.10; physician 12) is, in reality, a negative productivity ratio. This is because the amount of resources consumed, as measured by RVUs as a percent of the control group, is higher than the corresponding revenue distribution. Conversely, what may initially appear as a lower level of productivity (physician 3) results in a much higher level of productivity overall.

► Productivity vs. Profit

In Exhibit 6.12, you can see that a negative productivity (as seen in the fifth and tenth sets of bars as a value less than 1) does not always translate to negative profitability, as illustrated with physicians 5, 11, and 15. For this reason, care must be taken to determine the outcome of physicians whose productivity relationships are different from their profit values.

In closed panel arrangements or when revenue is fixed irrespective of the number and type of patients, work relative value units can be used to measure productivity and determine compensation.

PRODUCTIVITY USING WORK RELATIVE VALUE UNITS

There is a valid argument to be made about the bias of the previous methods with respect to fee schedule, billing, and collection issues. Nevertheless, because productivity must include both sides of the equation

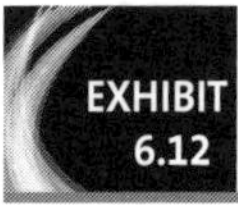

Ratio of Productivity vs. Profit/Loss

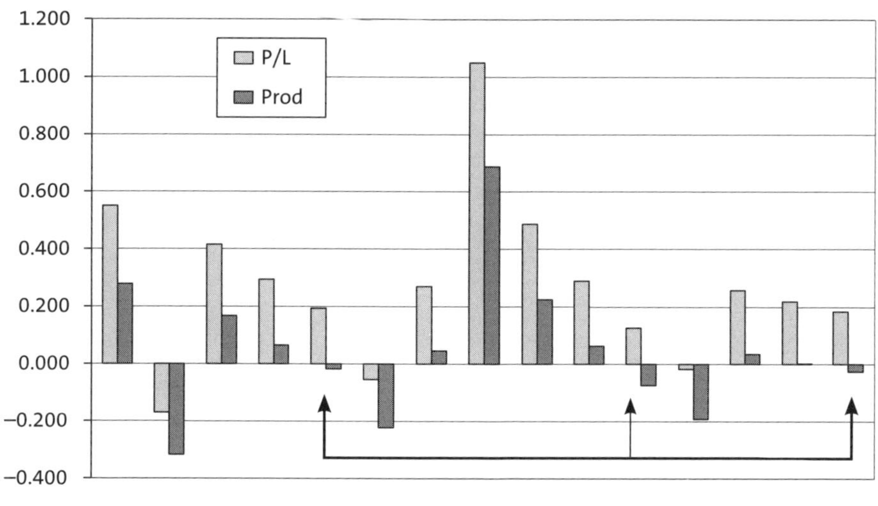

in a revenue-generating model, fair or unfair, both sides of the equation must be considered. In closed-revenue models, such as HMOs, prepaid closed panels, and similar models, work effort alone may be used to measure the relative productivity of a physician within a similar group. Because payment is based upon a group model or a flat negotiated contract amount and because revenue in this type of model is normally fixed, revenue-to-utilization ratios have little or no bearing on the productivity of the physician. Under these circumstances, productivity is measured solely by work effort or distribution of the work RVU component of the RBRVS.

Work Relative Value Unit Productivity Model

In the following example, an assumption of 1 FTE per provider is used, that is, each provider is considered to be a full-time employee who contributes the same number of hours to clinical patient care. A straight-line analysis shows the distribution of work effort for each provider based upon the work component of the RBRVS. In this example, you may find that physician 4 is able to process patients more efficiently or may treat a group of patients who require less time for evaluation, management, and treatment. In the case of physician 2, it could be that she or he is less efficient, spends more time with similar patients, or treats patients who are sicker or require a higher level of evaluation, management, and treatment. The latter, however, is rarely the case, because this would result in a higher work RVU per patient and therefore in a higher total RVU value and a higher ratio (see Exhibits 6.13 and 6.14). In this case, it would also be important to look at the number of patient visits for each physician and run a comparison between work effort and number of patients.

EXHIBIT 6.13 Work RVU (tabular)

ID	Work RVU	Ratio
1	1033.25	27.27%
2	785.14	20.72%
3	654.99	17.28%
4	1316.02	34.73%
TOTAL	3789.4	100.00%

EXHIBIT 6.14 Work RVU (graph)

Ratio

1

2

3

4

EXHIBIT 6.15 FTE Ratio (tabular)

ID	Work RVU	FTE	Ratio	n-FTE
1	1033.25	1.00	27.27%	27.27%
2	785.14	0.75	20.72%	27.63%
3	654.99	0.70	17.28%	24.69%
4	1316.02	1.00	34.73%	34.73%
TOTAL	3789.4	3.45	100.00%	28.99%

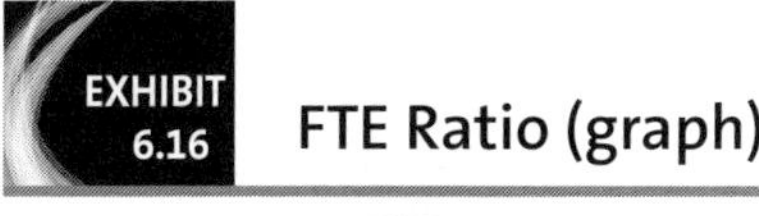
EXHIBIT 6.16 FTE Ratio (graph)

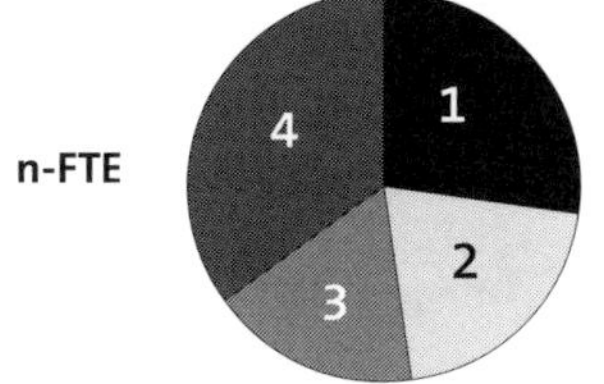

In the next example, assume that each provider is assigned a different FTE value, meaning that each provider works different hours and/or some contribute less time to the clinical patient care function than others (see Exhibits 6.15 and 6.16).

By dividing the ratio by the FTE value, the relationship can be normalized such that if a provider were, in fact, 1 FTE, his or her contribution would be as defined in the n-FTE column.

Revenue/Expense vs. Work Ratio

In the above example, the relationship of the work RVU can be compared with the relationship between the revenue to expense ratio developed earlier. This highlights the "work smarter, not harder" concept. In the case of provider 2, you can see that the relative contribution to the practice is greater than the work effort (work smarter) as opposed to that for provider 4, where the work effort is significantly higher than the overall contribution to the practice (work harder) (see Exhibits 6.17 and 6.18).

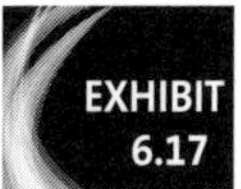
EXHIBIT 6.17 Revenue-to-Expense Ratio (tabular)

ID	Work RVU	WK Ratio	R/E Ratio
1	1033.25	27.27%	24.68%
2	785.14	20.72%	31.56%
3	654.99	17.28%	28.22%
4	1316.02	34.73%	15.54%
TOTAL	3789.4	100.00%	100.00%

EXHIBIT 6.18 Revenue-to-Expense Ratio (graph)

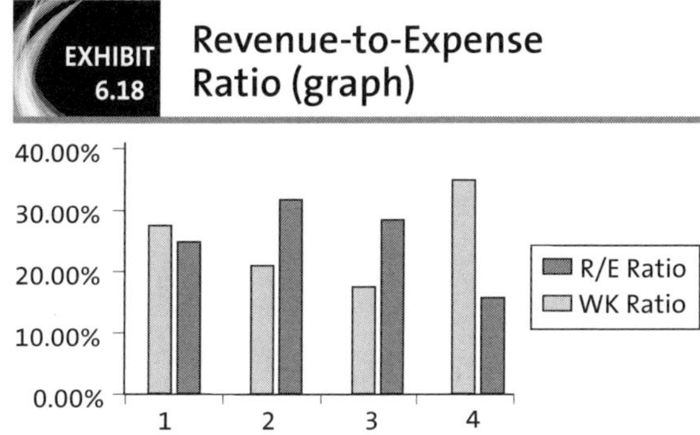

The question is, why is this happening? It could be due to coding, billing, and/or collection issues. It might also be due to the specific types of procedures the physician performs, although this is rarely the case in this type of model.

Work Effort vs. Profit/Loss Distribution

Exhibit 6.19 shows the comparison of each individual provider's work effort (measured as percent of total work RVUs) in relation to each provider's profit/loss as calculated in Exhibit 6.18. Note productivity for providers 5 through 9.

USING WORK RELATIVE VALUE UNITS TO ASSIGN FULL-TIME EQUIVALENT VALUES

Another value of the work RVU is in calculating or assigning FTE ratios for providers within the group. Again, it is important to remember that this is only viable as it relates to clinical work and does not take into account time spent in other activities, such as administration, research, teaching, or supervision.

EXHIBIT 6.19 Work Effort vs. Profit/Loss Distribution

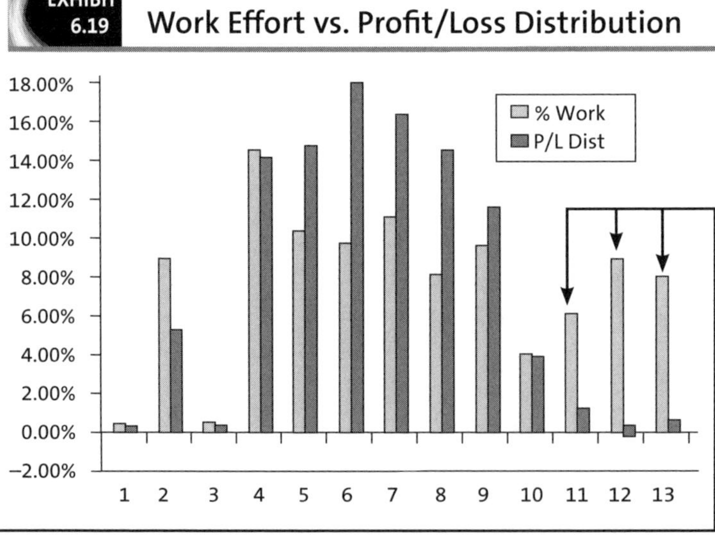

► Defining a Full-Time Equivalent

In the normal business environment, an FTE can be assigned by punch time or the actual time an employee reports working. The accepted FTE value for calculating salaries, wages, and benefits is 40 hours per week, or 2,080 hours per year, including vacation, sick, and personal time. For sales organizations, using time as a measurement of FTE ratios is less valuable because employee compensation is focused on production and the pay method is focused on commissions rather than straight salaries or hourly wage rates.

In healthcare, defining what constitutes 1 FTE is far more challenging because the actual punch time associated with physicians is harder to measure. In fact, today, with productivity becoming a defining issue, physician compensation looks more like that of a commissioned salesperson than a salaried laborer.

There are a few ways to define what constitutes 1 FTE, or full-time worker, within the practice. In a small practice, the task is really quite simple: poll the physicians to see who is defined as an FTE and use their RVU values as the average. Another method is based on the assumption that all employees contribute equally while working full time. In this case, divide the sum of the products of the individual work RVUs by the number of providers in the practice to get the defining average work RVU per FTE. Another method is to take the sum of the products of the providers' total work RVUs and divide by the stated number of FTEs. This may be determined by some administrative formula where the FTEs are claimed to be known.

Exhibit 6.20 represents a practice with eight orthopedic physicians. If all eight physicians worked an equivalent of full time at a base of 2,080 hours

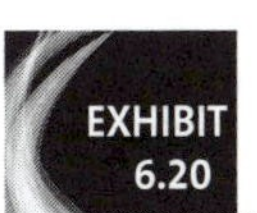

EXHIBIT 6.20 Example of How to Calculate Work RVU to FTE Relationship

Provider Name	Provider ID	Specialty	Work RVU
Doc 1	725	OS	5,019.12
Doc 2	726	OS	5,982.56
Doc 3	727	OS	6,904.16
Doc 4	728	OS	13,949.86
Doc 5	729	OS	6,000.80
Doc 6	734	OS	8,646.94
Doc 7	735	OS	13,797.70
Doc 8	736	OS	8,548.70
TOTAL			68,849.84

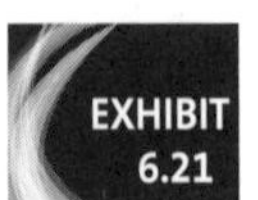

Example of How FTE Ratios are Calculated

Provider Name	Provider ID	Specialty	Work RVU	FTE Ratio
Doc 1	725	OS	5,019.12	0.65
Doc 2	726	OS	5,982.56	0.77
Doc 3	727	OS	6,904.16	0.89
Doc 4	728	OS	13,949.86	1.81
Doc 5	729	OS	6,000.80	0.78
Doc 6	734	OS	8,646.94	1.12
Doc 7	735	OS	13,797.70	1.79
Doc 8	736	OS	8,548.70	1.11
TOTAL			68,849.84	

per year, the median value of 7,726 could be used to approximate what constitutes 1 FTE provider. Exhibit 6.21 illustrates how this affects the providers.

Note that 50 percent (four physicians) are above 1 FTE and the other 50 percent are below 1 FTE. This makes sense because the median, which is same as the 50th percentile, is being used. But look at the variability between physicians. Only one or two physicians are really considered to represent what everyone would agree is the "typical" 1 FTE metric. For example, doc 3, doc 6, and doc 8 are considered the quintessential full-time workers. If the work values for these three docs are averaged, you get 8,033 work RVUs per 1 FTE (Exhibit 6.22).

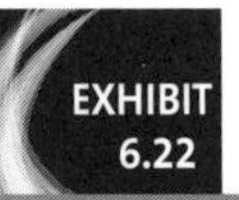

Using Selective Providers to Calculate 1 FTE Baseline

Provider Name	Provider ID	Specialty	Work RVU	FTE Ratio
Doc 1	725	OS	5,019.12	0.62
Doc 2	726	OS	5,982.56	0.74
Doc 3	727	OS	6,904.16	0.86
Doc 4	728	OS	13,949.86	1.74
Doc 5	729	OS	6,000.80	0.75
Doc 6	734	OS	8,646.94	1.08
Doc 7	735	OS	13,797.70	1.72
Doc 8	736	OS	8,548.70	1.06

Notice that there are still four physicians above and four below the 1 FTE; however, this time, there is a smaller variability (the standard deviation is a bit smaller), with a higher density around the 1 FTE mark. If doc 4 and doc 7 are considered to be the poster children for 1 FTE, everyone else would be part time! Use of this method involves a great deal of subjectivity and, in some cases, requires voting and consensus techniques to work. The key is to get a general acceptance before committing the results.

Irrespective of the methodology, it is important to establish a benchmark for an FTE. This is a primary consideration for compensation and benefits administration. Use of work RVUs for this purpose will provide a standard against which an equitable exchange can be measured and adjusted.

► Using Full-Time Equivalent Ratios for Compensation Calculations

Once an FTE is defined using an average RVU value, minimum requirements for salary and bonus calculations for the provider base can be assigned. The first step is to assign a minimum ratio of work RVUs as a percent of the average defined for 1 FTE. Let's assume that a practice uses 80 percent as this minimum value. If the practice reports an average RVU per FTE ratio of 7,500, then a provider would have to report at least 6,000 work RVUs per year, or 500 per month, in order to qualify for a base salary. If the provider falls short of that value, his or her salary for that month will be reduced by the difference between the average and the reported amounts. For the purpose of this example, let's assign a base salary of $150,000 per year, or $12,500 per provider per month. In order to qualify for the monthly salary amount, the provider must report 500 work RVUs. Also assume that provider A reports 450 work RVUs for the month of March. Calculated against the average of 625 work RVUs per month, this becomes 72 percent. The difference between this and the average is 28 percent, or $3,500. In this case, the provider's base salary for that month would be $9,000.

With respect to bonus distribution, the sample practice set a minimum benchmark of 90 percent, that is, in order to qualify for inclusion in the bonus pool, a provider would have to report at least 562.5 work RVUs (90 percent of the average monthly work RVU of 625). If a provider falls below this level, then she or he would not be able to share in the bonuses for that period.

Acuity factors not only help you solve the "my patients are sicker than others" issue but also identify potential evaluation and management coding issues for each provider.

In this example, a review period was defined as one month. However, periodization is up to the practice. My experience shows that many practices use quarterly rather than monthly periods to account for A/R days and rolling revenue calculations.

ACUITY FACTORING

In applying the acuity factor to physician productivity, you are attempting to accomplish two major tasks. The first is to quantify the "my patients are sicker than others" conundrum that plagues so many medical practices. The other is to determine whether potential evaluation and management (E/M) coding issues are skewing the acuity factor. In routine studies that use the acuity factor, comparisons are made to other markers, such as productivity, which help you to gain a better understanding of productivity anomalies that exist within the practice on a provider-by-provider basis.

In calculating physician productivity, you will use only the work RVU component. The first step, as defined in Chapter 2, is to total the number of procedures that have work RVUs and then divide by the total RVUs. Then, separate the E/M values from the non-E/M values in order to identify potential aberrancies with respect to E/M coding. This is done because coding for specific procedures is normally identified more accurately than coding for E/M visits.

When the total work acuity varies significantly among similar specialties in the same practice, it normally indicates coding anomalies.

Exhibit 6.23 shows the total acuity factor using work RVUs for all procedures for each provider in a cardiovascular practice. Although not exactly the same, the acuity factors for docs 1, 2, and 3 are relatively similar to the national average. However, the acuity factor for doc 4 varies significantly. This variance could be due to the fact that this provider

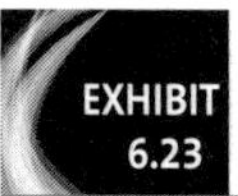

Comparison Using Total Work Acuity Factor

Acuity Using Work RVUs All Procedures

Provider	Practice	National	Variance
Doc 1	6.212	7.438	–16.48%
Doc 2	6.602	7.438	–11.25%
Doc 3	7.812	7.438	5.03%
Doc 4	4.143	7.438	–44.30%

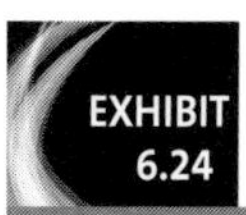

EXHIBIT 6.24 Work Acuity Factor for E/M and non-E/M Procedures

	Acuity Using Work RVUs All Procedures			Acuity Using Work RVUs E/M Procedures Only			Acuity Using Work RVUs non-EM Procedures Only		
Provider	Practice	National	Variance	Practice	National	Variance	Practice	National	Variance
Doc 1	6.212	7.438	−16.48%	4.312	1.655	160.59%	13.187	10.880	21.21%
Doc 2	6.602	7.438	−11.25%	1.514	1.655	−8.50%	10.667	10.880	−1.95%
Doc 3	7.812	7.438	5.03%	1.640	1.655	−0.91%	11.013	10.880	1.23%
Doc 4	4.143	7.438	−44.30%	0.981	1.655	−40.71%	10.788	10.880	−0.84%

sees patients who are outside the normal scope of the practice or it could indicate a different specialty within the group. However, in situations such as this, where there are multiple providers in the same specialty, a significant variance from the group normally indicates coding anomalies. Therefore, you will want to break the acuity out by E/M and non-E/M codes, as shown in Exhibit 6.24.

By breaking the acuity factor out by evaluation and management and non-evaluation and management, you can compare the ratios to identify evaluation and management coding problems or to quantify the complexity of the level of care required of the patient population for a specific provider.

As Exhibit 6.24 shows, doc 4 shows a significant variance from the national average when the acuity factor for the E/M codes only is compared, indicating at first glance that his patients do not require the same complexity of diagnoses and treatment as the patients for the other physicians. In essence, the values here would indicate that this provider's patients are not "as sick" as the patients seen by the other providers. Again, in this type of a situation, the severity of illness is normally not the reason for the variance. If you compare the acuity factors when using non-E/M codes, you see that doc 4 is at the national average and very close to the average for the other providers. This indicates that the non-E/M procedures the provider performs for his patients are "on the mark" when compared to the overall anticipated complexity of treating the entire patient population, further supporting the assumption that although his patients are "as sick" as the others, this provider has a tendency to under code E/M visits.

► Benchmarking with Acuity Factors

In Exhibit 6.25, there are three measurements for each provider. The first measures only the work effort. Exclusion of any reference to revenue or expense is not an accurate measurement of productivity alone, although

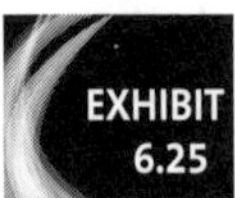

EXHIBIT 6.25

Comparison of Work, Acuity, and Productivity

Provider	Work Ratio	Acuity	Prod
Doc 1	1.09	1.37	1.05
Doc 2	0.83	0.82	1.34
Doc 3	0.69	0.64	1.19
Doc 4	1.39	1.14	0.66

it can be used to identify potential productivity issues within the practice and between providers. The next measurement of acuity does not measure productivity but can be used to adjust (or at least understand) the differences in work effort. Provid ers with a higher acuity ratio (indicating a more complex and resource-intensive patient base) would be expected to have a higher work ratio. The relationship between the two can be measured, adjusted, and normalized to determine potential problems with practice patterns and efficiency. Productivity measures the relationship between revenue and resource, giving a much truer picture of actual productivity. You could also add another column to show the relationship of each provider's profitability to that of the other providers if a cost analysis were first performed.

By graphing these factors, it becomes easy to spot anomalies within the productivity model.

Exhibit 6.26 allows for an overall analysis of these individual but related productivity issues.

For example, doc 1 does not show as high a work effort as doc 4, yet doc 1 has a higher acuity ratio, indicating that he or she may work more efficiently, all other things being equal. This is supported by the fact that doc 1 has a much higher productivity level than doc 4.

By segmenting the E/M from the non-E/M work acuity, you can often determine whether there are E/M-specific coding issues for a particular provider or measured entity. By comparing the provider's ratios to those contained within the national database, you can identify other potential practice anomalies. In looking at the ratio of E/M to non-E/M acuity factors (using the work RVU value), you would expect to see a higher ratio among primary care–type providers, such as those in internal medicine, family practice, and geriatrics, and a lower ratio among more specific specialty practices, such as the surgical disciplines.

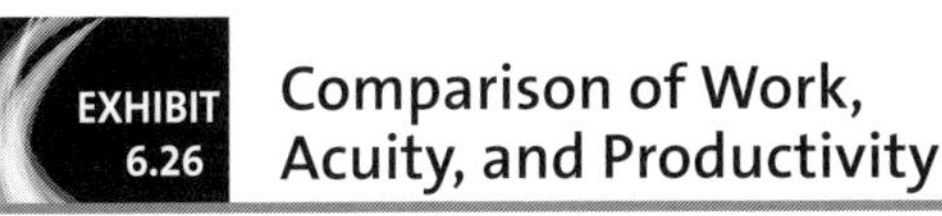

Comparison of Work, Acuity, and Productivity

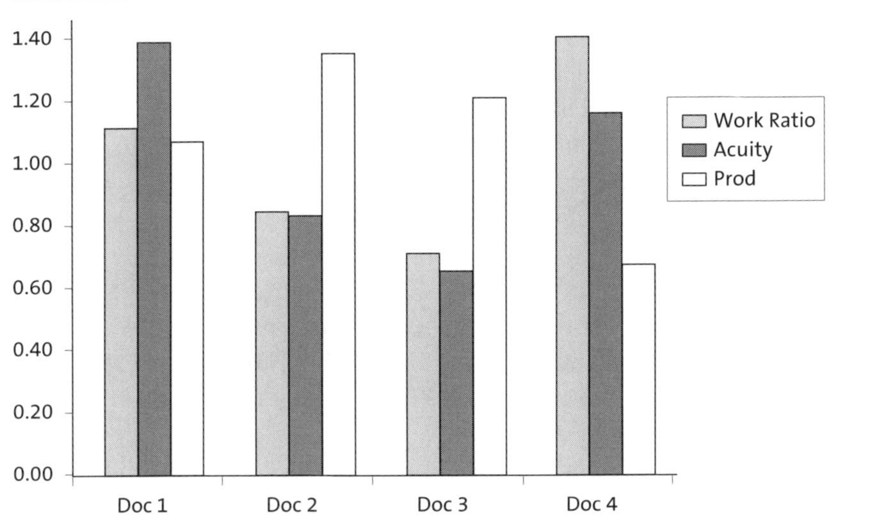

For example, if the ratio of the work E/M to the work non-E/M for a provider were higher than the national average for the same specialty, there might be a potential overcoding issue with respect to E/M codes. If the ratio were lower, then the opposite would likely be true. In this manner, you are able to first identify the potential skew of the acuity factor, which enables you to identify and correct coding problems.

COMPENSATION CASE STUDY

The following example describes a practice with 10 internal medicine physicians with approximate equality in seniority and an even distribution of payer mix among the patients. All are equal partners in the practice. The average of their salaries for the past three years (weighted as 25 percent, 25 percent, and 50 percent, respectively) was $175,000, with a range from $140,000 to $215,000. A decision was made to use the lowest salary, $140,000, as the base. This leaves $350,000 in the distribution pool. A decision was made to use profitability in order to distribute the pool to the individual providers.

Sample Salary Distribution

Profitability was calculated by first performing a procedural cost accounting analysis, calculating the cost per RVU and multiplying it by the number of RVUs assigned to each provider. Remember, this type of cost distribution is valid only in practices with a high degree of homogeneity. Then that amount was subtracted from the total revenue (gross receipts) to determine that physician's relative profit for the group. Provider 9 showed a loss for the year, and a decision was made to adjust the sample by that amount rather than deduct the loss from his base salary. To accomplish this, the loss amount ($2,588.64) was added to each provider's profit number. Then, each profit value was divided by the total profit/loss to assign a ratio based upon the entire group. To complete the cycle, the profit distribution percentage was multiplied by the pool of $350,000 for each provider and then added to his or her base salary amount, as shown in Exhibit 6.27.

Exhibit 6.28 illustrates the profit distribution after adjustment for the loss incurred by provider 9. If there are several negative producers, it is possible to eliminate them from the table and recalculate the profit relationships.

It is important to remember that this type of model is predicated on a rational normalization of financial systems within the practice with respect to coding, fee scheduling, billing, and collection.

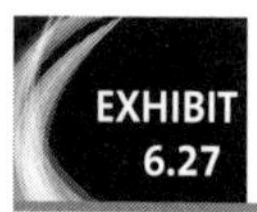

EXHIBIT 6.27 Sample Salary Distribution

ID	Revenue	RVUs	Cost	PL	Abs PL	P/L Dist	Base	Dist	Total
1	$303,823	6632.85	$256,134.25	$47,689.11	$50,277.75	5.67%	140,000	19,839	159,839
2	$528,168	10393.08	$401,339.23	$126,828.63	$129,417.27	14.59%	140,000	51,068	191,068
3	$424,455	7585.01	$292,902.81	$131,552.31	$134,140.95	15.12%	140,000	52,932	192,932
4	$444,019	7327.63	$282,963.90	$161,055.36	$163,644.00	18.45%	140,000	64,573	204,573
5	$459,470	8102.50	$312,886.01	$146,584.09	$149,172.73	16.82%	140,000	58,863	198,863
6	$363,381	6034.76	$233,038.26	$130,343.22	$132,931.86	14.99%	140,000	52,454	192,454
7	$371,224	6932.21	$267,694.14	$103,530.02	$106,118.66	11.96%	140,000	41,874	181,874
8	$186,789	4556.57	$175,956.55	$10,832.03	$13,420.67	1.51%	140,000	5,296	145,296
9	$244,794	6406.21	$247,382.16	−$2,588.64	$0.00	0.00%	140,000	0	140,000
10	$231,363	5854.92	$226,093.59	$5,269.61	$7,858.25	0.89%	140,000	3,101	143,101

EXHIBIT 6.28 Profit/Loss Distribution

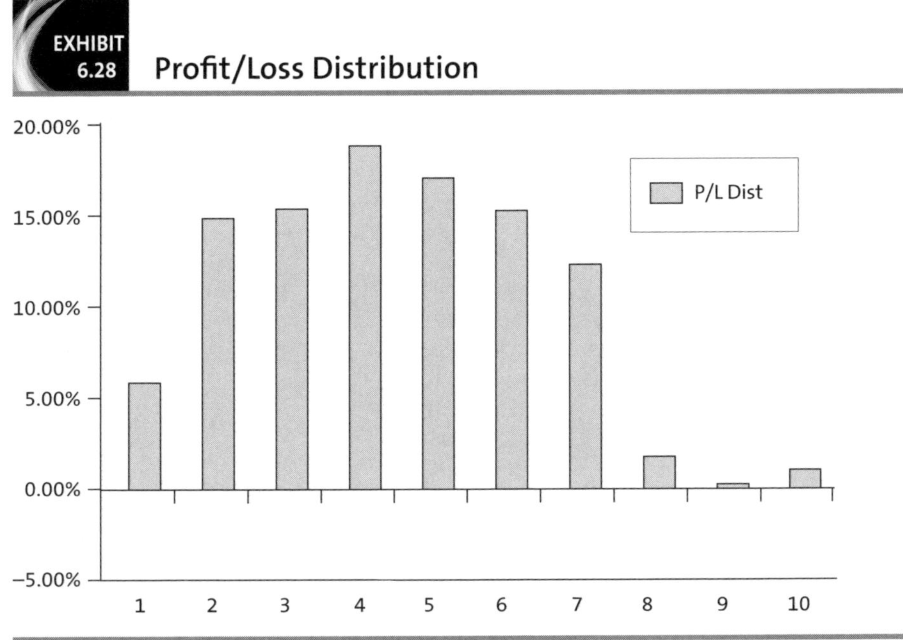

ADVANCED COMPENSATION ISSUES

As discussed previously, much of the distribution of costs in an even-spread model is predicated on the homogenous mix of markers within the practice. This works well with similar specialties, equality with respect to payer mix, rational distribution of administrative responsibilities, and similar conditions. This, however, is the exception and not the rule. In most practices, the dynamics are such that this equity in practice patterns is rare. Therefore, a more defining methodology for determining productivity, expenses, and profitability must be undertaken.

CASE STUDY USING COMPLEX COST MODELS

The following case study describes a six-physician practice made up of three family practice (FP) physicians and three internal medicine (IM) physicians. Exhibit 6.29 illustrates how expenses (costs) for each physician are defined using a simple spread-cost methodology of multiplying cost per RVU times the modifier-adjusted RVUs for each provider. In this case, cost per RVU was calculated using all applicable costs for the practice as a whole ($1,509,509), resulting in a value of $30.92.

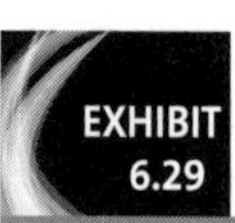

EXHIBIT 6.29 Cost Analysis Using Even Spread of Expenses

Specialty	Charges	Revenue	Collection	RVU Spread Cost
FP	$723,919	$340,876	47.09%	$264,105
FP	$747,332	$359,861	48.15%	$271,310
FP	$774,426	$349,055	45.07%	$248,613
IM	$408,121	$205,320	50.31%	$212,080
IM	$778,817	$367,009	47.12%	$247,315
IM	$772,190	$348,992	45.20%	$265,084
TOTALS	$4,204,805	$1,971,113		$1,508,509

Redistributing Malpractice as a Direct Cost

One issue facing the practice in this example was that of malpractice costs. The FP physicians had an annual malpractice bill of $17,000 each and the IM physicians' bill was $48,000 each year. Understandably, the FP physicians did not want to be saddled with the IM physicians malpractice cost. Consequently, the total malpractice amount of $195,000 was removed from the original expense amount and the new expense amount was used to calculate a new cost per RVU. Dividing the total RVUs into the new expense amount of $1,313,359 yields a cost per RVU of 26.92. As illustrated in Exhibit 6.30, the next step is to assign the malpractice cost as a direct expense to each physician, lowering the spread cost and changing the total expense while maintaining the total expense for the practice.

The overall result is to reduce the total cost assignment for the FP physicians while increasing the total cost assignment for the IM physicians.

Staff Resources as a Direct Expense

Having realized a negative effect from assigning the malpractice cost as a direct expense, the IM physicians were concerned over the way in which the expenses for the clinical staff in the office were being allocated. The argument was that the FP physicians had some staff members, in particular a nurse practitioner (NP), who were used almost exclusively by them. They countered that other staff, including an additional NP and a physician's assistant, were having their services utilized more by the IM physicians.

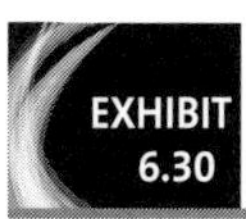

EXHIBIT 6.30 Using Malpractice as a Direct Expense

Specialty	Charges	Revenue	Collection	RVU Spread Cost	Malpractice	Total Cost
FP	$723,919	$340,876	47.09%	$229,939	$17,000	$246,939
FP	$747,332	$359,861	48.15%	$236,212	$17,000	$253,212
FP	$774,426	$349,055	45.07%	$216,451	$17,000	$233,451
IM	$408,121	$205,320	50.31%	$184,644	$48,000	$232,644
IM	$778,817	$367,009	47.12%	$215,321	$48,000	$263,321
IM	$772,190	$348,992	45.20%	$230,791	$48,000	$278,791
TOTALS	$4,204,805	$1,971,113		$1,313,359	$195,000	$1,508,359

As a result, the practice decided to do a full analysis of staff resources and to allocate expenses based upon utilization of those clinical staff members.

Allocation of Staff Resources

The first step was to identify the allocation of clinical staff resources. This was accomplished by showing the physicians a grid that identified each clinical staff member and having the physicians assign a utilization percent to each one based upon their perception of use. The simplest method was to first define which staff were utilized equally (16.67 percent) and then work backward from there (see Exhibit 6.31).

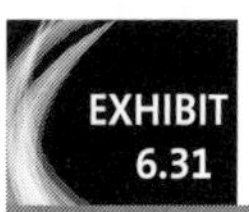

EXHIBIT 6.31 Distribution of Staff Resources Allocated by Physician

	1007	1009	1011	1004	1008	1010	Total
Mark	33.00%	33.00%	34.00%				100.00%
Nancy	16.67%	16.67%	16.67%	16.67%	16.67%	16.67%	100.00%
Jim	16.67%	16.67%	16.67%	16.67%	16.67%	16.67%	100.00%
Alice	25.00%		25.00%	25.00%	25.00%		100.00%
Jean				33.00%	33.00%	34.00%	100.00%
Cary	16.67%	16.67%	16.67%	16.67%	16.67%	16.67%	100.00%
Peter	16.67%	16.67%	16.67%	16.67%	16.67%	16.67%	100.00%
Louise					100.00%		100.00%
Margaret	16.67%	16.67%	16.67%	16.67%	16.67%	16.67%	100.00%

Distribution of Expenses

The next step was to assign the expense for each staff member, based on the resource allocation results, to each physician as a direct expense (Exhibit 6.32). This is calculated by multiplying the percent utilization assigned in the previous step by the total compensation value for each employee. In this case, the numbers were estimated. However, it is important to consider all expenses related to each employee that would be considered a practice expense, such as medical insurance, payroll contributions, and similar expenses.

Assigning Allocation as a Direct Expense

Once the final costs have been calculated for each physician, these values are first deducted from the total expenses used to calculate the cost per RVU. In this case, you would subtract the $388,800 in clinical staff expenses from the $1,313,359 used to calculate the prior value, resulting in a spread expense amount of $925,522. Dividing this by the number of calculated modifier-adjusted RVUs, the cost per RVU goes from 29.62 to 18.97, substantially reducing the spread cost now assigned to each provider. The difference is assigned as a direct expense to each physician commensurate with the allocation of the costs listed in Exhibit 6.33.

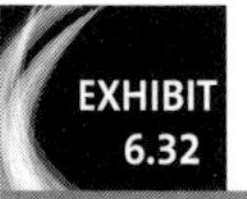

Distribution of Expenses for Clinical Staff Based on Allocation

	1007	1009	1011	1004	1008	1010	Total
Mark	$10,230	$10,230	$10,540	$—	$—	$—	$31,000
Nancy	$10,833	$10,833	$10,833	$10,833	$10,833	$10,833	$65,000
Jim	$5,667	$5,667	$5,667	$5,667	$5,667	$5,667	$34,000
Alice	$13,750	$—	$13,750	$13,750	$13,750	$—	$55,000
Jean	$—	$—	$—	$21,450	$21,450	$22,100	$65,000
Cary	$4,667	$4,667	$4,667	$4,667	$4,667	$4,667	$28,000
Peter	$4,667	$4,667	$4,667	$4,667	$4,667	$4,667	$28,000
Louise	$—	$—	$—	$—	$52,000	$—	$52,000
Margaret	$5,000	$5,000	$5,000	$5,000	$5,000	$5,000	$30,000
TOTALS	**$54,813**	**$41,063**	**$55,123**	**$66,033**	**$118,033**	**$52,933**	**$388,000**

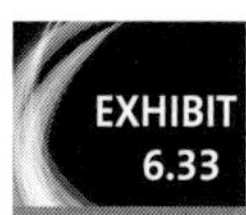

Redistribution of Costs Based on Allocation of Staff Resources

Specialty	Charges	Revenue	Collection	RVU Spread Cost	Malpractice	Staff Allocation	Total Cost
FP	$723,919	$340,876	47.09%	$162,036	$17,000	**$54,813**	$233,849
FP	$747,332	$359,861	48.15%	$166,456	$17,000	**$41,063**	$224,519
FP	$774,426	$349,055	45.07%	$152,531	$17,000	**$55,123**	$224,654
IM	$408,121	$205,320	50.31%	$130,117	$48,000	**$66,033**	$244,150
IM	$778,817	$367,009	47.12%	$151,735	$48,000	**$118,033**	$317,768
IM	$772,190	$348,992	45.20%	$162,636	$48,000	**$52,933**	$263,569
TOTALS	$4,204,805	$1,971,113		$925,511	$195,000	**$387,998**	$1,508,509

Distributions Based on Excess Capacity

Another issue that was raised by the IM physicians dealt with the distribution of expenses related to excess capacity. Their logic was that they spent much less time in the office than the FP physicians did because they spent time admitting, discharging, and visiting with hospital-based patients. Their idea was to perform a time study in order to determine what percent of their time was spent in the office compared with that of the FP physicians. The objective was to divide the excess capacity based on this definition of actual time spent in the office. This raised some serious concerns about the intent of a group practice. It was decided that rather than distributing excess capacity based on productivity or RVUs, it would be split equally among the providers.

Defining Excess Capacity

The first step was to define the value of the excess capacity for the practice. This was accomplished by calculating an optimum visit level and factoring that by the current visit level. It was decided that the practice had a 10 percent excess capacity factor. Fixed costs (or what was defined as facility cost) were calculated as $377,127. Ten percent of this, $37,713, was defined as excess capacity. Equal distribution was accomplished by dividing by the number of physicians in the group (6), for a total direct assignment of costs of approximately $6,285 per physician (see Exhibit 6.34).

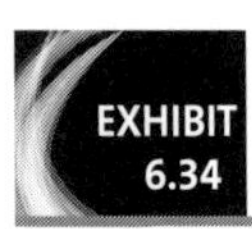

EXHIBIT 6.34 Distributions Based on Excess Capacity

Specialty	Charges	Revenue	Collection	RVU Spread Cost	Malpractice	Staff Allocation	Excess Capacity	Total Cost
FP	$723,919	$340,876	47.09%	$155,433	$17,000	$54,813	**$6,285**	$233,532
FP	$747,332	$359,861	48.15%	$159,673	$17,000	$41,063	**$6,285**	$224,022
FP	$774,426	$349,055	45.07%	$146,316	$17,000	$55,123	**$6,285**	$224,724
IM	$408,121	$205,320	50.31%	$124,815	$48,000	$66,033	**$6,285**	$245,133
IM	$778,817	$367,009	47.12%	$145,552	$48,000	$1,18,033	**$6,285**	$317,870
IM	$772,190	$348,992	45.20%	$156,009	$48,000	$52,933	**$6,285**	$263,228
TOTALS	$4,204,805	$1,971,113		$887,798	$195,000	$387,998	**$37,713**	$1,508,509

As in previous steps, it is necessary to readjust the spread RVU cost. This is done by subtracting the $37,713 from the spread expense amount and recalculating the new cost per RVU, which, in this case, is now $18.20. Then, the excess capacity direct cost is added as a line item to get the total cost assigned to each physician.

► Recalculating Profit/Loss by Provider

The above represents one solution for one practice. It is important to understand that these types of applications can differ significantly from one practice to another and sometimes within one practice from one year to another.

Once a consensus has been reached and a viable cost model has been finalized, you then recalculate the profit/loss amounts by provider in order to complete the compensation model. Exhibit 6.35 defines this distribution

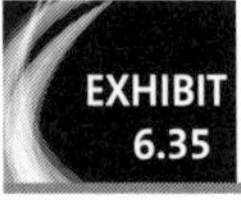

EXHIBIT 6.35 Profit/Loss Distribution Using Nonallocated Expenses

Provider ID	Specialty	Charges	Revenue	Collection	Cost	Profit/Loss	Profit/Loss
1007	FP	$723,919	$340,876	47.09%	$264,105	$76,771	**16.60%**
1009	FP	$747,332	$359,861	48.15%	$271,310	$88,551	**19.14%**
1011	FP	$774,426	$349,055	45.07%	$248,613	$100,442	**21.71%**
1004	IM	$408,121	$205,320	50.31%	$212,080	$(6,760)	**−1.46%**
1008	IM	$778,817	$367,009	47.12%	$247,315	$119,694	**25.87%**
1010	IM	$772,190	$348,992	45.20%	$265,084	$83,908	**18.14%**

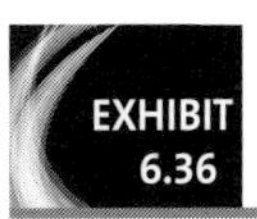

EXHIBIT 6.36 Profit/Loss Distribution Using Allocation of Direct Expenses

Provider ID	Specialty	Charges	Revenue	Collection	Cost	Profit/Loss	Profit/Loss
1007	FP	$723,919	$340,876	47.09%	$233,532	$107,344	**23.20%**
1009	FP	$747,332	$359,861	48.15%	$224,022	$135,839	**29.36%**
1011	FP	$774,426	$349,055	45.07%	$224,724	$124,331	**26.88%**
1004	IM	$408,121	$205,320	50.31%	$245,133	$(39,813)	**–8.61%**
1008	IM	$778,817	$367,009	47.12%	$317,870	$49,139	**10.62%**
1010	IM	$772,190	$348,992	45.20%	$263,228	$85,764	**18.54%**

as it originally stands, without redistribution using direct expense calculations.

Exhibit 6.36 illustrates the significant differences in total expenses assigned to each physician by using a direct-expense allocation approach.

By comparing these two tables, you see that although the total profit/loss remains the same, the way in which this is allocated by physician changed significantly. Overall, the FP physicians benefited from this methodology while the IM physicians did not. Although this may seem inequitable at first, it is important to note that the IM physicians received a base salary that was approximately 35 percent higher than that of the FP physicians. Also, although this redistribution did not bring the total compensation to a par value, it did help to mollify many of the compensation problems that existed prior to the application of this methodology.

Recalculating Compensation

The final step is to recalculate compensation using the profit/loss distribution provided earlier in conjunction with the bonus pool established by the practice. First you need to deal with the issue presented by provider 1004. He was the only one to show a loss using both unallocated and allocated methods. As discussed earlier, there are two ways to deal with this; the practice decided to simply eliminate this physician from the tables, allowing a natural redistribution of the profit/loss percentages.

Again, it is prudent to look at the comparisons between allocated and unallocated compensation methods. Exhibit 6.37 shows the distribution

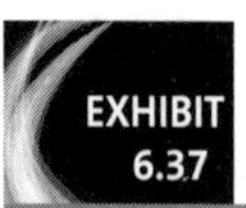

EXHIBIT 6.37 Compensation Based on Unallocation of Expenses

Provider ID	Specialty	Profit/Loss	Base Salary	Bonus	Total Comp
1007	FP	16.36%	$140,000	$57,247	**$197,247**
1009	FP	18.87%	$140,000	$66,031	**$206,031**
1011	FP	21.40%	$140,000	$74,898	**$214,898**
1008	IM	25.50%	$175,000	$89,254	**$264,254**
1010	IM	17.88%	$175,000	$62,569	**$237,569**

of salary plus bonus (total compensation) using the spread-cost method in which costs were not allocated by exception.

You can see that provider 1004 is not included in Exhibit 6.37, yet the bonus amount ($350,000) remains constant. Notice that this method increases the variance inequity in compensation between the two groups.

In Exhibit 6.38, you see that although the IM physicians maintain a higher base salary, bonus distribution (which is based solely on the allocated profit/loss model) helps to achieve a more reasonable parity between the two groups. Although some may consider the IM physicians to be entitled to earn more as a result of their specialty designation, they also have a higher expense associated with that designation. This is a common issue in multispecialty practices, and it is important to remember that parity needs to be measured in all areas. Where there are both primary care and surgical specialties, malpractice premium costs alone can vary by a factor of 15 and sometimes even more.

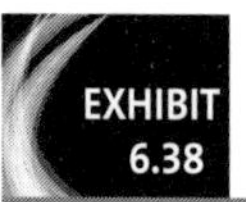

EXHIBIT 6.38 Compensation Based on Allocation of Direct Expenses

Provider ID	Specialty	Profit/Loss	Base Salary	Bonus	Total Comp
1007	FP	21.37%	$140,000	$74,780	**$214,780**
1009	FP	27.04%	$140,000	$94,630	**$234,630**
1011	FP	24.75%	$140,000	$86,613	**$226,613**
1008	IM	9.78%	$175,000	$34,232	**$209,232**
1010	IM	17.07%	$175,000	$59,746	**$234,746**

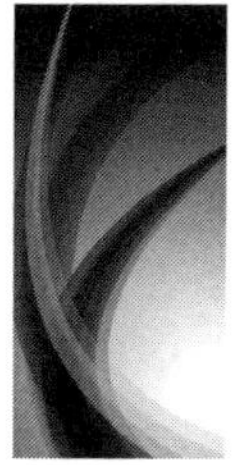

CHAPTER 7

Fee Schedule/ Reimbursement Analysis

The fee schedule is the single most important financial tool in the medical practice. As such, it is essential that you analyze the fee for every procedure code/modifier combination so as not to minimize the financial impact that 80 percent of the codes will have on your practice.

The fee schedule, sometimes referred to as the charge master, is the single most important financial tool within the medical practice. As with any other business, the fees a practice charges reflect the value of the products and services delivered. When you strip away the clinical component of a medical practice, it is, in reality, just another business. And like any other business, a medical practice is concerned with expenses, employees, insurance, taxes, and just about every other business-related issue.

It is surprising that so many practices create and maintain their fee schedules without a solid understanding of the basic methodology that is used or the potential impact a poorly derived fee schedule can create. There is a broad array of methods that practices employ; some that follow logical paths and others that are tied to models that favor the payers rather than the physicians. Physicians should subscribe to a philosophy of independence, their decisions should be based on sound economic and market-based principles, and they should not be held hostage to payers.

EXISTING FEE SCHEDULING METHODS

Research suggests that there are six basic methods most medical practices use to establish and adjust their fees. These methods are described in the following paragraphs.

► Medicare Fee Schedule Amount

Although more timely in its research than other methods, the Medicare fee schedule (MFS) is subject to significant political and financial pressures that override the validity of the research used to develop it. Not only is the conversion factor (CF) affected by annual financial factors, the practice expense and malpractice expense relative value unit (RVU) values are also subject to change based on reasons other than effective and appropriate research. Although the MFS should not be used to develop and adjust a commercial fee schedule, it can be used as a factor of the minimum amount that should be established for the practice.

► Usual, Customary, and Reasonable Values

Usual, customary, and reasonable, having been at the center of many controversies and lawsuits, still dominates the market when it comes to pricing and contract negotiations.

The use of usual, customary, and reasonable (UCR) values has been at the core of pricing and negotiation contracts for managed care providers for many years. The UCR values, if calculated correctly, provide a statistical analysis of the amounts providers from around the country charge for their services. It is not a secret that this amount can vary significantly based on specialty designation and geographical location. As such, UCR calculations should take these two factors into consideration. Unfortunately, many of the UCR tables that are published do not necessarily use appropriate statistical methodologies and they lack analytical data points, such as variances and sample error, which are critical when assessing the value of the information. In recent years, the Office of Attorney General for the State of New York, led by then Attorney General Andrew Cuomo, found that the most prominent of UCR databases, the Ingenix database, was seriously flawed and subject to considerable conflict of interest. It is owned, maintained, and updated by UnitedHealthcare. As such, it is important to know and understand the methodology and data sets used in creating a UCR database in order to avoid being deceived, as so many were with the Ingenix data.

► Relative Value Studies

The resource-based relative value scale (RBRVS) was never designed to approximate the fair value for services and procedures reported by a medical provider. Rather, it was designed to measure the associated consumption of resources. In its early stages, the scale didn't even do a very good job of that. However, after 20 years of improvement, RBRVS is not a bad model for measuring expenses within a practice. If used from a cost-plus-markup perspective, it works quite well. However, when used only in relation to the CF, it is basically the same as using the MFS, only with a variable CF. For example, if you increase the CF by 10 percent, you have increased the fee for each procedure by 10 percent. This is easy to do, but consider that this method may increase the charge for procedures that are already priced too high while not increasing the charge enough for procedures that are priced too low. Although using RVS is a good way to establish a fee for a new procedure or to adjust a fee for an existing procedure (in order to profile the fee schedule), it doesn't always have a strong or supportable econometric foundation, which, from a defensibility standpoint, should be your goal.

Surveys and Published Lists

The question to ask when considering a published fee schedule is, where did the data originate from? In most cases, the data are obtained from UCR surveys, health maintenance organization pricing, Civilian Health and Medical Program of the Uniformed Services data sets, and other noncommercial payer groups. In effect, these lists combine charges with what the potentially lower-paying payers are paying and then simply extrapolate those data into low, medium, and high payment amounts based upon percentile ratings. Irrespective of what they may claim, none of the companies that sell these lists know, with zip code granularity, exactly what physicians are charging or being paid for all of their services. Second, have you ever wondered how timely these data can be? Even the most aggressive research organizations, such as the MGMA–ACMPE and the American Medical Association, are usually one year behind the data stream in producing their research reports. Considering granularity, some claim to be able to produce a fee schedule by specialty by zip code. There are approximately 70 specialties recognized by the Centers for Medicare & Medicaid Services (CMS) and more than 40,000 zip codes in the United States. This would mean that these companies would need data on 2.8 million fee schedules to build those profiles, a number that simply does not exist.

Flat Increases

Flat increases are a favorite among many financial types who look at the balance sheet for the practice and determine that they need to increase fees to make up for an increase in costs. The problem is that the increase in fees represents an increase in charges, not collections. For those procedures with charges that already exceed a logical maximum, this will only increase write-offs and disallowances. For charges that are significantly lower than reasonable, the slight increase will more than likely fall short of bringing the charge into a competitive yet profitable zone.

► Asking Other Physicians

Not only is it illegal to ask other physicians about what they charge, it is stupid (can I say that here?). Imagine basing the fee that is charged for a procedure on what another practice charges, having no clue as to what methodology they use to adjust their fees. Although a medical practice faces issues that are similar to those of other businesses, each is a unique entity unto itself, with unique financial, operational, and personnel considerations. Establishing or adjusting a fee by asking other physicians is like cheating off someone's test without knowing whether they have the right answers. More accurately, it's like reading a good copy of a bad X-ray. Enough said.

Basing your charges on what another physician charges is not only illegal, it's just plain stupid (can I say that here?).

In what follows, fee scheduling will be reviewed from six basic perspectives:

- The process of benchmarking using RBRVS and Medicare
- Comparative analyses using national and local average fees
- Econometric models, such as price plus markup
- Acuity factors, which measure the level of complexity of the services and procedures provided to a patient population
- Global analytical modeling using categorical CFs
- Volumetric methods, such as fees based on hourly and work RVU values

Absent some logical method, the practice is left with two alternatives: guessing and asking other physicians. The former lacks judgment and good sense to such a degree that it does not even bear discussion and the latter, in the broadest stroke of interpretation, is most likely illegal. If not illegal, it reflects a less intelligent approach than just guessing. In fact, basing fees on those of another practice, whose methodology may also be in question, that may also have "guessed," reduces the probability that guessing may achieve a reasonable fee schedule by an order of magnitude.

Physicians should become aware of the need for constant review and evaluation when considering adjustments to their fee schedule. If the practice is losing money on a particular procedure, doing more of that procedure or betting on the "make it up in volume" philosophy will not work. If the practice realizes that the fee for a particular procedure is higher than what is reasonable, it is just as important to consider reducing that fee as it is to consider increasing a fee for a procedure that is below a reasonable threshold.

A proper and thorough fee schedule analysis is much more than raising fees, it may have nothing to do with fee adjustments at all. Raising fees is easy, and anyone without the benefit of specific skills or knowledge can do it with the stroke of a pen or the tap of a key on the keyboard. But raising fees does not address the issue of moving the medical practice toward integration with accepted and viable business models.

Establishing and maintaining a fee schedule for a medical practice can be as easy as calculating a ratio of Medicare reimbursement. It can also be as complex as incorporating real-time market econometric dynamics, such as the consumer price index (CPI), Medicare economic index (MEI), labor rate fluctuations, and other related financial indicators. For most practices, reality falls somewhere in the middle.

The primary purpose of the information being provided in the fee schedule is to assist the practice in reaching a level of profitability that allows it to thrive within a market and to deliver high-quality healthcare to its patients consistently. Without this, quality suffers and, consequently, so does the community being served.

WHAT IS A FEE SCHEDULE?

It is important to first define what constitutes the practice's fee schedule. According to CMS, "a fee schedule is a complete listing of fees used by Medicare to pay doctors or other providers/suppliers. This comprehensive listing of fee maximums is used to reimburse a physician and/or other providers on a fee-for-service basis. CMS develops fee schedules for physicians, ambulance services, clinical laboratory services, and durable medical equipment, prosthetics, orthotics, and supplies."

Looking at this, it may be easier to define what a fee schedule is *not*. A fee schedule is *not* simply a database that assigns a charge to each procedure and/or service delivered by a physician. Also, a fee schedule is *not* a knee-jerk reactionary instrument that is used to validate an amount a payer claims to be reasonable. A fee schedule is a concise tool that gives patients, payers, regulators, and reviewers a clear picture of how the practice defines the value of its services. A well-developed and well-maintained fee schedule sends a signal that the practice is market sensitive, fiscally responsible, and organizationally sound.

FEE SCHEDULE PHILOSOPHY

It's a simple concept; your charges should be balanced between the value of your services and what the market can bear.

It is difficult to say what drives the decisions healthcare professionals make when developing their fee schedules. Historically, fee schedules were constructed based on an idea of cost and profitability. A physician provided a service for a patient, billed the insurance company, and got paid; this model seems draconian today. Within the past two decades, however, fee schedule methodologies have been reduced to a race to control write-offs and disallowances; a measure of the unreasonableness of the payer side. In essence, practices have settled on a fee schedule that is based on what payers are willing to reimburse.

The fee schedule philosophy advanced here is that practices should adopt a methodology that takes advantage of accurate internal and external data. Under the UCR model, which looks like it may be around for a while, future contract reimbursement levels will be based largely on charge levels of today. Establishing charges on what another entity/payer views as fair may very well limit the ability of the practice to negotiate accurate fees that cover practice costs in the future.

METHODOLOGICAL CONSIDERATIONS

Within the fee scheduling methodology, there are several variables that must be considered. Some variables are directly related to (and in control of) the practice. These variables may include expenses, CFs, total compensation, and, to some degree, payer mix. Some variables such as market dynamics, malpractice costs, population fluctuations, and supply costs may well be outside of the practice's control. Developing a fee schedule for each practice should remain independent of specific charges used by other practices within the same market area. It is important to ensure that the methodology used depends upon practice-specific variables in order to minimize the risks of antitrust actions. This approach also ensures that a practice's fee schedule is based on its own internal functionality, not on the fee schedule from another practice, which may or may not have a similar business model.

Additionally, by using large aggregate data sets for benchmarking, the practice is able to compare its charge structure with that of its peer group. Although comparative data should not be used as a sole determinant for the fee schedule, it is helpful for understanding the value other physicians within the same specialty place on the services provided to their patients.

BENCHMARKING FEES

A benchmark is a standard against which something can be measured or judged. If the practice is unable to calculate market value for any single procedure code or group of procedure codes, it is acceptable for a practice to benchmark its fees against an external set of standards.

In this first step, you begin to establish benchmarks against external metrics that, to some, may feel like the old way of doing business but, in fact, represent a model for setting reasonable and logical limits. Use of benchmark methods may prove to be the most complex of what will be discussed here; however, these methods also tend to be the easiest to defend, making them a powerful tool for negotiating profitable contracts.

Although not considered even a reasonable fee schedule by many, the MFS is used to ensure that charges are not below the MFS's allowable amount or, for many practices, below a ratio of the MFS allowable.

The RBRVS, which is the basis behind developing the MFS, is used to establish and compare the CF levels for each code and, more importantly, each coding category. Global CF values help you to "see" the bigger picture as it relates to overall charge levels within homogenous groups. For example, comparing the mean CF for all surgical procedures for general surgeons against the same metric for a general surgery practice would give the practice a high-level view of the overall charge structure for its surgical procedures.

The Physician/Supplier Procedure Summary Master File (P/SPSMF) contains 100 percent of all claims submitted to Medicare during a calendar year. This database includes 5 billion claims containing every billable procedure code submitted to CMS represented by nearly every physician in every specialty in nearly every region of the United States. And because nearly 95 percent of practices submit their "usual and customary" (retail) charges to Medicare, the P/SPSMF is an excellent data source to use when determining average charge levels by national and state aggregates for each procedure code by specialty.

Competitive Factor

After taking financial aspects into consideration, competition drives fees in nearly every industry. Practices that are more competitive, either by specialty or location, may want to be more sensitive to the fees they charge. This is particularly true for evaluation and management (E/M) codes because they are often "shopped" by patients in highly competitive markets. For the purpose of the fee analysis, competitiveness is broken down into five levels, from most competitive (level 1) to least competitive (level 5). In the most competitive state, fewer procedures will be recommended for increase; for those procedures that do meet the criterion, the increase amount will be less. The levels are described as follows:

- Level 1 is for those practices that choose to be very competitive in their pricing. These are usually primary care practices located in an urban area of a highly populated city, competing with many other physicians for basic primary care business.
- Level 2 is for those practices that choose to be conservatively competitive. Although they recognize the need to adjust their fees reasonably, they may be in a competitive market or may offer only general primary care services, such as a walk-in center or urgent care center.
- Level 3 is for those practices that choose to maintain an average competitive presence. They want their fees to fall in the median range for similar types of physicians in their area.
- Level 4 is for those practices that choose to be somewhat less competitive than those in level 3. This will result in more procedures being flagged for increase and a slightly higher increase for those flagged.
- Level 5 is for those practices that choose to be noncompetitive in their pricing structure. At this level, the increases will be much more significant than in lower levels, as will be the amount of the increases.

Establishing the Charge Thresholds

The minimum charge threshold (MinCT) is measured as a ratio of the MFS and enables the practice to determine the point at which the fee for a procedure may be considered below an accepted minimum amount.

In essence, the threshold acts as the floor for the fee schedule model. Although a fee for a procedure that is below this threshold may trigger a review, when considering competitiveness, it does not always indicate that the fee will be adjusted.

The CF amount is calculated by multiplying the MinCT ratio for each competitive category by the current Medicare CF. Exhibit 7.1 illustrates how this would work. In this case, the CY 2012 CF of 34.0376 is used.

The maximum charge threshold (MaxCT) is measured as a ratio of the MFS. The MaxCT enables the practice to determine the point at which the fee for a procedure may be considered above the maximum amount. In essence, the MaxCT is the ceiling for the fee schedule model. Although the fee for a procedure above this threshold may trigger a review, when considering competitiveness, it does not always indicate that the fee will be adjusted.

The CF amount is calculated by multiplying the MaxCT ratio for each competitive category by the current Medicare CF. Exhibit 7.2 illustrates how this would work using the CY 2012 Medicare CF of 34.0376.

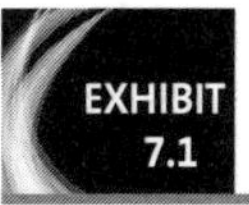

Example of Minimum Charge Threshold Calculations

Competitive Factor	Minimum Charge Threshold	CF Amount
Very competitive	1.1250	38.2923
Somewhat competitive	1.3125	44.6744
Average competitive	1.5000	51.0564
Not very competitive	1.6875	57.4385
Not competitive at all	1.8750	63.8205

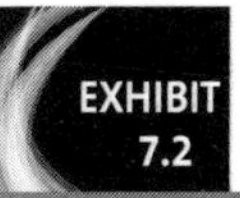

Example of Maximum Charge Threshold Calculations

Competitive Factor	Maximum Charge Threshold	CF Amount
Very competitive	3.00	102.1128
Somewhat competitive	3.50	119.1316
Average competitive	4.00	136.1504
Not very competitive	4.50	153.1692
Not competitive at all	5.00	170.1880

It is important to remember that the charge thresholds are established to trigger an event only, that of closely reviewing the fee for a procedure against other benchmarks. It is also important to note that just because the fee for a procedure meets one of the above criteria, it does not necessarily mean that the fee will be automatically adjusted.

DATA ELEMENTS

In order to perform a fee schedule analysis, the following are required:

- Fee schedule
  - Procedure code with modifier, if any
  - Commercial fee amount
  - Annual (or other periodized) frequency
- Physician fee schedule database
  - Contains all RVUs, geographic practice cost indices, and critical usage information
- P/SPSMF
  - P/SPSMF produced by physician billing group of CMS
- Local econometric data
- CPI, MEI, and local, regional, and national information

With this data in hand, you can now perform a proper fee analysis.

► Building the Spreadsheet

To begin, build a worksheet that will serve as the basis for many of the different fee analysis models that will be discussed here. Start by listing the procedure code in the first column, the modifier (if any) in the next column, the fee charged to commercial or private payers (reasonable fee) in the next column, and the frequency for the data period being analyzed in the next column.

The next step is to determine the gross charges for each procedure code. To do this, multiply the frequency for each code by the fee and place this number in the next column.

In order to develop both CF and MFS comparisons, the total geographically adjusted RVU for each code and the total RVUs based upon frequency calculations must be included.

To obtain the MFS amount, multiply the geographically adjusted RVU by the Medicare CF. Next, calculate the CF for each procedure code, or record, by dividing the charge by the adjusted total RVU. Finally, calculate the distributed CF by category. To do this, divide the grand total fee amount by the grand total RVU amount for each major code category. Exhibit 7.3 provides a sample of a completed table.

Adjusting the Fees

To identify procedures that may need a fee adjustment, first identify those fees that are under the MFS allowable amount. This is done by comparing the CF for each procedure code with the current year's Medicare CF. If the CF for the code falls below the Medicare CF for the current year, it is identified as being below that MFS allowable amount, or the amount published by CMS for a practice in a given geographic location. The next step is to identify codes where the cost of providing the service exceeds

First and foremost, you should take a look at procedures where your charge is less than the Medicare allowable.

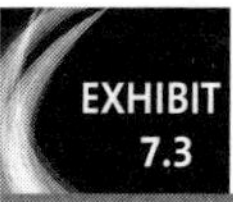

EXHIBIT 7.3 Example of Completed RBRVS Table

Code	Fee	TPY	Tot Fee	RVU	Tot RVU	MFS-NF	CF
10060	$70	59	$4,130	2.07	122.41	$70.59	33.74
10140	$55	33	$1,815	2.51	82.98	$85.55	21.87
11040	$95	919	$87,305	1.01	928.19	$34.36	94.06
11050	$35	40	$1,400	0.81	32.44	$27.59	43.16
11422	$300	12	$3,600	3.53	42.34	$120.05	85.02
11720	$35	61	$2,135	0.74	45.14	$25.18	47.30
11730	$115	358	$41,170	1.77	632.41	$60.10	65.10
11750	$379	208	$78,832	3.76	781.77	$127.88	100.84
20550	$37	42	$1,554	1.93	81.22	$65.80	19.13
28090	$250	10	$2,500	9.16	91.61	$311.68	27.29
28126	$510	103	$52,530	8.67	892.50	$294.81	58.86
28286	$775	313	$242,575	9.76	3,055.36	$332.12	79.39
28296	$1450	409	$593,050	18.45	7,548.05	$627.89	78.57
28298	$1410	403	$568,230	16.70	6,730.77	$568.24	84.42
29540	$29	116	$3,364	0.94	108.60	$31.85	30.98
29580	$375	9	$3,375	2.47	22.23	$84.04	151.82
TOTALS			$1,687,565		21,198.02		79.61

the collection amount. This is accomplished by reviewing results of the cost accounting analysis. *This is only valid if the cost per RVU is less than 120 percent of the Medicare CF.* If the cost per RVU for the practice, as calculated in the cost accounting analysis, is greater than 120 percent of the Medicare CF, the practice, in most cases, has expense problems, not fee problems, and simply raising the fee for a procedure will not result in an associated increase in reimbursement.

Next, identify those codes below the MinCT. This is based on a CF that is calculated as a ratio of the Medicare CF. Procedure codes in your table that have a CF that is less than this value are identified and included in the analysis for possible fee adjustments later. Finally, identify groups that have fees in excess of the MaxCT, where the CF is in excess of the MaxCT ratio. When you are finished, a completed table may look like Exhibit 7.4.

Note that the letter Y has been placed in the fields associated with codes that met one or more of the criteria outlined above. The practice, of course, may use any method to identify codes that meet or fall within

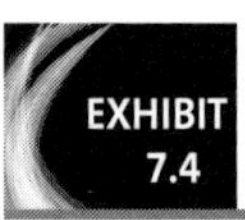

Example of Table with Criteria Columns Included

Code	Fee	TPY	Tot Fee	RVU	Tot RVU	MFS-NF	CF	MFS	MinCT	MaxCT
10060	$70	59	$4,130	2.07	122.40	$78.63	33.74	Y	Y	
10140	$55	33	$1,815	2.51	82.97	$95.29	21.87	Y	Y	
11040	$95	919	$87,305	1.01	928.19	$38.28	94.06			
11050	$35	40	$1,400	0.81	32.43	$30.73	43.16		Y	
11422	$300	12	$3,600	3.53	42.34	$133.72	85.02			
11720	$35	61	$2,135	0.74	45.14	$28.04	47.30		Y	
11730	$115	358	$41,170	1.77	632.40	$66.95	65.10			
11750	$379	208	$78,832	3.76	781.76	$142.44	100.84			
20550	$37	42	$1,554	1.93	81.22	$73.29	19.13	Y	Y	
28090	$250	10	$2,500	9.16	91.61	$347.18	27.29	Y	Y	
28126	$510	103	$52,530	8.67	892.50	$328.39	58.86			
28286	$775	313	$242,575	9.76	3055.36	$369.94	79.39			
28296	$1450	409	$593,050	18.45	7548.05	$699.39	78.57			
28298	$1410	403	$568,230	16.70	6730.77	$632.95	84.42			
29540	$29	116	$3,364	0.94	108.59	$35.48	30.98	Y	Y	
29580	$375	9	$3,375	2.47	22.23	$93.61	151.82			Y
TOTALS			$1,687,860		21198.01		79.62			59.72

the criteria. In Exhibit 7.4, for example, procedure code 10060 has been identified as having a fee below both the Medicare CF and the MinCT. Code 29580 is identified as having a fee that is greater than the designated MaxCT. This does not mean that the fee will automatically be reduced; however, reducing the fee may be an option based on reimbursement from all payers.

► Determine the Fee Adjustment Amount

Although the determination of how much to adjust a fee can get quite complex, for most practices it will be based on an understanding of and experience with the economy, both nationally and in a specific geographic location. Following are several sources that may be considered when determining the percent adjustment:

- Categorical CFs
- MEI
- Medical component of the CPI
- Inflationary indices (local and national)
- Specific relevant data (i.e., the U.S. Department of Housing and Urban Development to determine increases in lease amounts or the U.S. Department of Wage and Labor to determine the average salary by specific Standard Industrial Classification code)

If the information or indicators are unknown, they can be accessed via the Internet. For example, by typing "consumer price index" in the search field of any Internet search engine, volumes of material regarding these financial metrics can be located.

Using the mean conversion factor by category—that which is calculated from your own charges—ensures that your fee schedule is, at least, consistent.

► Establish Resource-Based Relative Value Scale–Based Adjustment Amount

For procedures that are below the MFS, below the MinCT, or above the MaxCT, the goal is to utilize the mean CF for that code category. If the mean CF for the code category is below the minimum charge amount established earlier, the minimum charge amount could be used. In the same manner, if the mean CF for the code category is above the maximum charge amount that was previously established, the maximum charge amount could be used.

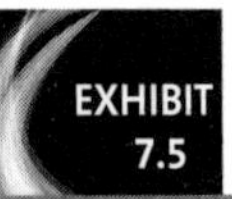

Example of Completed Fee Schedule Analysis Table

Code	Fee	TPY	RVU	MFS-NF	CF	MFS	MinCT	MaxCT	New Fee
10060	$70	59	2.07	$78.63	33.74	Y	Y		$165.19
10140	$55	33	2.51	$95.29	21.87	Y	Y		$200.20
11040	$95	919	1.01	$38.28	94.06				
11050	$35	40	0.81	$30.73	43.16		Y		$64.56
11422	$300	12	3.53	$133.72	85.02				
11720	$35	61	0.74	$28.04	47.30		Y		$58.92
11730	$115	358	1.77	$66.95	65.10				$125.32
11750	$379	208	3.76	$142.44	100.84				$413.00
20550	$37	42	1.93	$73.29	19.13	Y	Y		$153.98
28090	$250	10	9.16	$347.18	27.29	Y	Y		$729.40
28126	$510	103	8.67	$328.39	58.86				$638.17
28286	$775	313	9.76	$369.94	79.39				
28296	$1450	409	18.45	$699.39	78.57				
28298	$1410	403	16.70	$632.95	84.42				$1,536.48
29540	$29	116	0.94	$35.48	30.98	Y	Y		
29580	$375	9	2.47	$93.61	151.82			Y	$300.00

Based on the work completed so far, a fee analysis table may look something like Exhibit 7.5.

► Calculate the Net Financial Impact

The financial impact to the practice is normally less than the difference between the new fee and the current fee times the frequency. This is due to collection based on payer mix. Unless the fee for the procedure is below that of Medicare, an increase in a fee will not result in an increase in Medicare reimbursement. The same holds true for most managed care.

One simple way to calculate the financial impact is to multiply the gross impact (variance by frequency) times the average collection percent for the practice. A more detailed calculation will take into account the payer mix that would be affected (primarily true indemnity or commercial fee-for-service payers). For the latter, calculate the percent collection expected by the expected frequency and total, as shown in Exhibit 7.6.

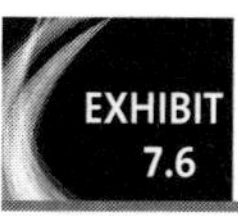
EXHIBIT 7.6

Example of Collection Estimates by Line and Total

Code	Fee	TPY	MFS	MinCT	New Fee	Variance	Gross	Net
10060	$70	59	Y	Y	$165	95	$5,616	$2,672
10140	$55	33	Y	Y	$200	145	$4,792	$2,280
11040	$95	919						
11050	$35	40		Y	$65	30	$1,183	$563
11422	$300	12						
11720	$35	61		Y	$59	24	$1,459	$694
11730	$115	358						
11750	$379	208						
20550	$37	42	Y	Y	$154	117	$4,913	$2,338
28090	$250	10	Y	Y	$729	479	$4,794	$2,281
28126	$510	103			$638	128	$13,202	$6,281
28286	$775	313			$775	0	$0	$0
28296	$1450	409						
28298	$1410	403		Y	$1,536	126	$50,970	$24,252
29540	$29	116	Y	Y	$75	46	$5,283	$2,513
29580	$375	9						
TOTALS							$92,211	$43,874

COST ACCOUNTING

In many businesses, fees are established based on a standard cost-plus-markup methodology. This is quite common in retail stores. For example, a hardware store may want a 70 percent markup on certain building products. Determining the fee for such products is easy, just add 70 percent to the cost of the product. Many small businesses, especially sole proprietorships, fail because the owner doesn't understand the concept of this method. A lawyer who charges $500 per hour doesn't make that amount; the $500 is the gross revenue before expenses, taxes, and similar costs. If a consultant wants to earn, say, $50 per hour, he or she can't charge $50 per hour; the consultant needs to charge $50 per hour above and beyond the cost of delivering the service.

Cost-plus-markup is a very common method for establishing charges. In healthcare, however, the problem is not what you charge, it's what the payer is willing to pay.

Note here that it's critical to know the cost of your product or service; this has been a holy grail among healthcare providers for as long as I can remember. Think about the basic concept here: do you know what your hard cost is to perform an office visit? Or to do a minor surgical procedure? Or to see a patient as a follow-up to a major surgical procedure? The fact is that the overwhelming majority of practices don't know these costs. How can you intelligently sign a managed care contract that promises a certain fee for a certain procedure when you don't know if that fee is above or below your cost? The answer is, of course, you can't.

From the perspective of a fee analysis, you can use costs either on an individual basis to determine contract profitability and/or to calculate a global fee schedule based on this cost-plus-markup method. The first step is to determine your costs, which is a lot easier than most people think.

First build a basic RBRVS table similar to Exhibit 2.1. Remember to include only those procedures that have an RVU value. Those that don't are usually supplies, such as drugs and casting material. It is relatively easy to develop a fee for these types of materials; because you know what you paid for them, adding a markup is as simple as adding your markup ratio to the cost.

For RVU-based procedures, multiply the RVU value times the frequency and then divide this into the total expenses for the data period. For example, if a practice were to report 18,000 RVUs during the data period and their expenses (minus the cost of non-RVU supplies) were $615,600, they could calculate $34.20 as the cost per RVU ($615,600 divided by 18,000 RVUs). This allows them to do two things: calculate the average cost per procedure and create a cost-plus-markup fee schedule.

The former is a relatively simple process; multiply the cost per RVU times the RVU value for the procedure, which is easily found in the public domain. For example, a mid-level outpatient consult (code 99243) has an associated non-facility unadjusted total RVU of 3.43. Multiply this times the cost per RVU ($34.20) to get a hard cost of $117.30. Remember, this is the cost based on what you included in your total expenses. Inclusion of physician compensation represents total costs including what the physician earns.

It is a bit simpler to use this model to create or maintain a fee schedule than to approach it from a line-item basis. Take the cost per RVU, add a markup, and multiply this number times the RVU value for the individual code. For example, let's say that you want to have a 100 percent markup over your expenses. Double the cost per RVU and you have a charge-per-RVU value of $68.40. Multiply this times the RVU for the individual procedure and you have the new fee. If you extend this to the above example, the new fee for the 99243 procedure is $234.60 (total RVU of 3.43 times the charge-per-RVU of $68.40).

It is important to remember that just because you bill using a particular fee doesn't mean that you will be paid the amount you charge. This rarely, if ever, happens. If you are considering the use of a charge-based methodology, it is very important to have a handle on your average collection ratios by payer type in order to ensure that, in any case, your costs do not exceed collections.

TIME-BASED CALCULATIONS

Lawyers do it. Accountants do it. And many consultants do it. What do these professionals have in common? They charge by time. Charging by a unit of time is an age-old method of fee scheduling. Notice that I didn't say "charging by the hour." For those of you who have dealt with an attorney recently, you may have noticed that they charge by small increments, such as 15-minute or even 6-minute intervals of time. So, here's the $64 thousand question: if other professionals can do it, why can't physicians? And the answer is, they can!

Many professionals such as accountants, lawyers, and consultants charge based on time. Why not physicians?

There are basically two ways to implement this. The first is to simply pick an hourly amount out of the air, say, $400. The second is to incorporate existing data, such as cost, charge, or revenue per hour, to create a benchmark for these types of calculations.

Picking a rate out of the air doesn't mean that there isn't some link to reality, it just means that you aren't considering existing internal data to do so. For example, let's say that local attorneys are getting $400 an hour for services rendered. Most physicians have spent more time in school and in training than the typical attorney, so a unit charge of $400 per hour would certainly pass muster as a reasonable amount.

Converting this hourly rate to a charge for a procedure, however, is a little trickier than it would be for an attorney. The reason is that the physician's services are more redundant. Physicians do the same things over and over, and although diagnosis and treatment issues are huge, the charge is based on the procedure, not the final outcome. Also, physicians want to maintain the same charge for the same procedure for all payer models, and this requires, in effect, figuring out the average time spent for each procedure. This means that some kind of standard reference is needed in order to define the amount of time. This reference can exist in one of two ways: the practice can create it or the practice can use an established standard. To create the reference from scratch, the practice would have to record the amount of time spent for each procedure with a sample size large enough to create a mean (or median) time that is statistically significant. The other option would be to use the Relative Value Scale Update Committee (RUC) time study, which is readily available on the CMS Web site.

Regardless of the standard, the model will be the same. However, for the following example, the RUC study is used. The methodology is actually very simple; multiply the number of mean minutes for the procedure times the charge per hour (in this case, reduced to charge per minute).

Following from above, let's look at an example for this. The practice has decided on a rate of $450 per hour. Dividing by 60, this comes out to $7.50 per minute. The RUC study reports the mean number of minutes for this procedure (code 99213, office visit, established) as 23. Multiply the $7.50 per minute by the reported 23 minutes to get a charge of $172.50. Because this is a common procedure and the practice is sensitive to office visit charges, it probably isn't a surprise that this seems excessive. Some practices, wanting to be sensitive to the needs of their community, reduce the value for E/M codes in accordance with internal cultural standards. This always needs to be considered.

If you run the same analysis for a surgical code, say 49000 (exploration of abdomen), the charge would be the charge per minute ($7.50) times the number of minutes (304), which equals $2,280.

The data source references are the same here as with the above example. The difference is that the practice has existing data supporting a charge-to-time ratio. For example, the practice reported (for a particular physician) 2,080 work hours with total charges of $500,000. Dividing the charges by the work hours, you get approximately $240 per hour (or $4 per minute). Going back to code 99213, the fee would be $92 ($4 per minute times 23 minutes). For the surgical procedure example, the fee would be $1,216 ($4 per minute times 304 minutes).

Use of work RVUs results in a bit of an "end run" around the time-to-charge ratio, but it is effective as a methodology. The work RVU is calculated primarily based on the number of minutes reported in the RUC study, which provides a powerful relationship between charge per work RVU and charge per (RUC) minute. The difference is that the work RVU includes both (RUC) time as well as effort. As such, some consider it a more accurate metric.

Back to the above example, let's take the physician who reported the $500,000 in gross charges for a given year. During that same data period, the physician reported 5,656 work RVUs. Divide the gross charges by the work RVUs and you get an average charge-to-work RVU ratio of $88.40.

Moving into the analysis, multiply the work RVUs reported for code 99213 (0.92) by the ratio of $88.40 to get a fee of $81.38. For the surgical code 49000, the fee would be $1,100 ($88.40 times 12.44 work RVUs).

The only caveat here is that when establishing the fee using work RVUs only, the practice is discounting the relative cost associated with these procedures. In some cases, this can be significant. The practice may want to consider using the total RVU rather than just the work RVU because, in the current RBRVS model, the practice expense RVU is based on the same RUC time.

GLOBAL CONVERSION FACTORS

Conversion factors are dollar values that are used to convert the RVU value for a procedure into a fee. For example, the Medicare CF for 2012 was 34.0376 and procedure code 99213 had a total (nongeographically adjusted) RVU of 1.68. Multiplying the two together, the Medicare par nonadjusted allowable amount is $57.18.

The previous paragraph describes how to calculate the Medicare allowable using the Medicare CF. Let's apply a little algebra and use the practice's current fee, then divide by the RVU to get the CF for a code (or group of codes) for the practice. For example, if the practice charges $92 for 99213, dividing by the total RVU of 1.68, the CF is $54.76. By accumulating this data by major code category, the practice is then able to calculate the mean CF.

For our purposes, let's calculate mean CFs for the following categories:

- Surgical: 10000 through 69999
- Radiology: 70000 through 79999
- Laboratory and pathology: 80000 through 99999
- E/M: 99201 through 99499
- Medicine: 90000 through 99999 (excluding E/M codes)
- Healthcare Finance Administration Current Procedural Coding System II: prefix A through prefix V

For most practices, it is easiest to use the median CF for each category. The median, also referred to as the 50th percentile, is simply the middle value in a list of values. To calculate the median CF for the surgical group, the practice would list the individual CF for each surgical procedure in a spreadsheet, sort the procedures in ascending order by CF, and then take the middle value as the median. If there is an even number of values, the average of the middle two would be used. For example, if the practice listed nine CF values in the spreadsheet, they would use the fifth as the median, with four values below and four values above the fifth. If there were 10, take the average of the values in position five and six would be used.

Let's take a practice that has gone through this scenario. They have calculated their surgical CFs and come up with a median of 100 for the surgical group. The median for all physicians with their specialty from the national database is 111. In this case, the practice's surgical CF is around 90 percent of the national average, indicating that its global charge model is below that of its peers. Exhibit 7.7 gives some examples of global CF values by category for different geographic locations.

Remember, the global CF calculations don't necessarily pinpoint issues with individual codes. Rather these calculations point the practice to other methods, such as average charge comparisons, to help you understand the comparative relationships by individual code.

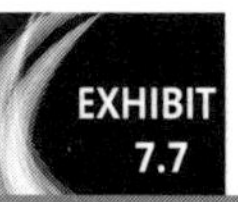

Examples of Global Conversion Factors by Category

State	Carrier Number	Pricing Locality	Surgical	Radiology	Pathology	Medicine	E/M	Average
MD	901	1	90.59	104.68	77.94	79.81	58.08	76.93
MD	901	99	75.17	83.74	92.98	69.08	51.88	65.21
MD	−1	−1	86.52	98.94	80.87	76.90	56.27	73.67
ME	31142	3	86.05	105.80	98.33	65.71	56.10	71.61
ME	31142	99	78.26	95.11	106.55	62.03	53.46	67.04
ME	−1	−1	81.56	99.39	103.30	63.66	54.54	68.94
MI	953	1	69.64	90.85	95.90	75.64	52.27	66.44
MI	953	99	70.90	81.00	77.27	71.04	51.11	63.72
MI	−1	−1	70.34	86.10	86.51	73.54	51.72	65.12
MN	954	0	74.18	75.17	61.40	64.06	58.11	65.32
MN	−1	−1	74.18	75.17	61.40	64.06	58.11	65.32

CHARGE DATA COMPARISONS

Once a new fee schedule has been established, recommendations should be compared with the average charge levels for those codes, for both national and state averages. This can be done using data that are specialty-diagnostic or for the specific specialty of the practice conducting the analysis. These data are also compiled from the P/SPSMF. Remember, the majority of physicians and practices submit their commercial charges to Medicare, as opposed to just the Medicare allowable. Therefore, the charge database contains reasonable charges; simply put, the database is huge. If a practice chooses to calculate the averages itself, it should use total charges submitted and do so only for unmodified codes because philosophies for charging for modifiers remain inconsistent.

In using these data, be careful not to make adjustments to the recommended new fees based solely on average charge levels, at least don't do so expecting to get a one-to-one ratio of reimbursement. However, these data may be used to assess the fees within the community, defined by both specialty and geographic boundaries. It can be assumed that the charge data for all practices, all claims, and all specialties are the average charge data representing just that—the average for all practices. Therefore, if the practice is unique (e.g., cancer center, tertiary facility), it would be

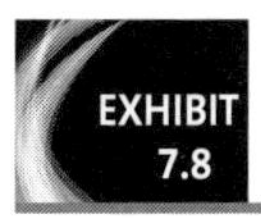

EXHIBIT 7.8 Example of Comparison of Practice Fees to Benchmark Fees

Code	Description	Fee	National Median	National Mean	State Mean	Below National Mean	Below State Mean
10060	Drainage of skin abscess	$70.00	$120.00	$130.50	$122.74	1	1
10140	Drainage of hematoma/fluid	$55.00	$150.00	$176.24	$109.56	1	1
11055	Trim skin lesion	$35.00	$44.74	$50.68	$55.81	1	1
11720	Debride nail, 1-5	$35.00	$38.45	$49.05	$45.66	1	1
11730	Removal of nail plate	$115.00	$103.63	$112.49	$116.64	—	
11750	Removal of nail bed	$379.00	$250.00	$265.28	$204.33	—	
20550	Inj tendon sheath/ligament	$37.00	$100.00	$109.99	$91.05	1	1
28090	Removal of foot lesion	$250.00	$610.00	$659.33	$551.09	1	1
28126	Partial removal of toe	$510.00	$567.30	$604.78	$505.55	1	
29540	Strapping of ankle and/or ft	$29.00	$48.63	$51.99	$53.87	1	1

reasonable to expect the practice's charges to be higher than average. The same holds true for the other side of the spectrum.

The only time that these data should be used to adjust a fee is when there are major variances between the practice's fee schedule amount and the average charges. The charge database is really no more than a tool to understand the value that other providers place on the work they do. Exhibit 7.8 illustrates a sample fee comparison.

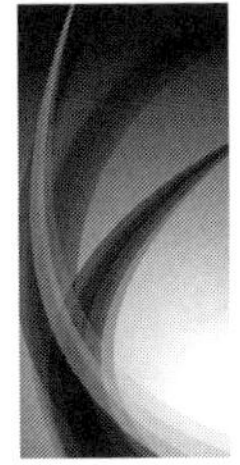

CHAPTER 8

Applications to Managed Care

Here lies the great inequity in the field of healthcare; the insurance company, loaded with all the tools and resources necessary to guarantee themselves a profit, versus the typical medical practice, struggling to keep up and trying to compete with an empty toolbox. The problem is that when the only tool you have is a hammer, pretty soon everything starts to look like a nail.

It goes without saying that the transition from fee-for-service to other payment methodologies has been a painful process for many medical practices. In fact, it's been painful for the healthcare industry as a whole. Most physicians just want to practice medicine, and the financial component involved in the practice of medicine necessitated that many physicians become as adept at business as they are at science. The good news is that it has helped many physicians to understand the importance of oversight. The bad new is that it is a lot more expensive than many thought it would be, from opportunity cost for the provider to increases in staff and technology to manage the billing and collections processes. In the past, the practice simply treated a patient, billed for the service, and got reimbursed by an insurance company. Now the practice must know which company they are going to bill in advance, understand each of their policies, track payment for a specific fee schedule, and ensure that what they are getting paid is correct under that specific contract. Managing the wide array of managed care options, plans, and agreements can be a nightmare for some practices. In many cases, these agreements are signed without an understanding of the financial impact they could have on the practice. The question becomes, why bother spending money on an attorney to work on the wording of a contract if you are not certain that the contract will be profitable? In previous chapters, we examined some ways to apply the resource-based relative value scale (RBRVS) to managed care. For example, in Chapter 4, you learned how to determine whether the fee schedule being offered was reasonable based on procedural costs and break-even fees. In Chapter 7, you learned how to position your fees for future consideration and how to optimize your revenue through analysis of modifier relationships. In this chapter, the focus is on how to determine the financial and resource impact of managed care contracts and how to determine profitability prior to signing on the dotted line.

MANAGED CARE AND THE MEDICAL PRACTICE

The potential for profitability or disaster within the managed care contract lies less in the wording than it does on the pragmatic mathematics used to determine the viability of the fee schedule.

This chapter focuses on a new and more analytical way to examine RBRVS applications to managed care contracts. Much of this information is based on the ability to calculate levels of utilization of procedures and services and how this relates to staffing, the physical plant, and clinical capabilities. Often a practice takes on a new contract only to later realize that they were simply not ready to handle the influx of patients. Or even worse, a practice gears up for a near invasion only to realize that most of the new "contract patients" are existing patients and very few are new to the practice. In the following sections, you will learn how to:

- Calculate utilization per thousand
- Project changes in visit level based on the number of insured lives
- Apply variable costs for capitation and other managed care organization models
- Calculate total and variable contract costs
- Calculate the practice's existing cost per member per month (PMPM)

UTILIZATION CALCULATIONS

When calculating utilization per thousand, you are determining how many of a certain procedure and/or service will be provided for every thousand active patients within the practice. The results of this analysis will be used to project patient visit volume, contract cost, and other contractual component projections.

Data Requirements

To begin, build a basic spreadsheet that contains the fee, relative value unit (RVU) components, and annual (or periodized) frequency for each procedure code/modifier group (Exhibit 8.1). It is necessary to know the total number of active patients (not patient visits) and to have already performed a cost analysis by calculating cost per RVU for both total and variable expenses.

Calculate Utilization per Thousand

The first step in calculating utilization per thousand patients is to determine the number of active patients. Then, divide the frequency of the procedure by the number of active patients in the practice and multiply by 1,000. Data in Exhibit 8.2 are based on a total active patient base of 9,043. Each frequency is divided by 9,043 and then multiplied by 1,000. For example, procedure code 99203 in Exhibit 8.2 indicates utilization per thousand of 99.75. This means that for every 1,000 new (or existing) active patients, you can expect to report 99.75 new mid-level office visits (99203).

Whether the practice is experiencing excess, optimal, or maximum capacity can make a huge difference in which expense model is to be used to calculate contract cost.

Assign Cost

The next step is to assign a unit (procedural) cost for each line item (code group). To accomplish this step, a cost accounting analysis must have been performed and a cost per RVU value established. You can either copy the cost from the cost accounting results or multiply the appropriate RVU

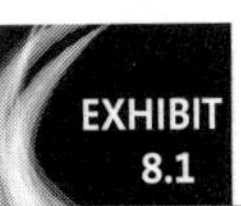
EXHIBIT 8.1 Collecting the Basic Data

Code	Description	Fee	Freq
10060	Drainage of skin abscess	$129	75
17000	Destroy benign/premlg lesion	$146	410
45330	Diagnostic sigmoidoscopy	$243	29
58150	Total hysterectomy	$1432	40
59025	Fetal non-stress test	$137	253
99203	Office/outpatient visit, new	$151	902
99213	Office/outpatient visit, est	$97	15,543
99243	Office consultation	$191	24

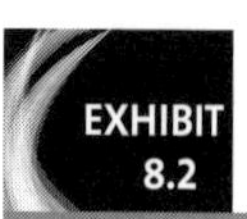

Calculating Utilization per Thousand

Code	Description	Fee	Freq	Utilization per Thousand
10060	Drainage of skin abscess	$129	75	8.29
17000	Destroy benign/premlg lesion	$146	410	45.34
45330	Diagnostic sigmoidoscopy	$243	29	3.21
58150	Total hysterectomy	$1432	40	4.42
59025	Fetal non-stress test	$137	253	27.98
99203	Office/outpatient visit, new	$151	902	99.75
99213	Office/outpatient visit, est	$97	15,543	1,718.79
99243	Office consultation	$191	24	2.65

value for each code by the category cost per RVU. In Exhibit 8.3, the total cost per RVU has been calculated at $32.23 and the variable cost per RVU has been calculated at $9.46.

Variable Cost Calculation

Variable costs include the supplies and materials that are directly related to the patient visit. In calculating the variable cost per RVU, first calculate the total variable expenses related to patient visits for the practice. Then, divide this by the total number of calculated modifier-factored RVUs for

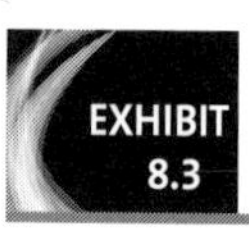

Assigning Costs

Code	Description	Fee	Freq	Utilization per Thousand	Total Cost	Variable Cost
10060	Drainage of skin abscess	$129	75	8.29	$79.12	$23.22
17000	Destroy benign/premlg lesion	$146	410	45.34	$51.99	$15.26
45330	Diagnostic sigmoidoscopy	$243	29	3.21	$103.39	$30.35
58150	Total hysterectomy	$1432	40	4.42	$784.91	$230.38
59025	Fetal non-stress test	$137	253	27.98	$35.35	$10.38
99203	Office/outpatient visit, new	$151	902	99.75	$82.38	$24.18
99213	Office/outpatient visit, est	$97	15,543	1,718.79	$45.26	$13.28
99243	Office consultation	$191	24	2.65	$103.57	$30.40

the same entity. For example, if the variable costs for this practice totaled $156,842 and the total RVUs were calculated at 16,570.5, you would divide the variable costs by the RVUs to get a cost per RVU of $9.46. To get the cost per procedure, multiply the variable cost per RVU times the RVU value for that group.

MEASURING VISIT CAPACITY

A practice faces three types of capacity issues. Excess capacity is a condition that exists when there is more space and staff than there are patients. In an excess capacity situation, the practice may not be seeing enough patients to cover its expenses. If they are seeing enough patients, the number of patients may be just above the minimum. Excess capacity can occur when a physical plant is bigger than it needs to be; when a practice is substantially overstaffed; or, as is common, in a new practice where the patient visit load has not yet normalized. In situations of excess capacity, the practice is often losing money because the cost per patient visit exceeds the reimbursement per patient visit. In these situations, the practice normally cannot afford variable-cost contracts and must base reimbursement on total costs instead.

If a new contract will result in visits that exceed maximum capacity, it is critical to work the additional costs required to manage the contract back into the contract amount.

Optimal capacity exists when the facility and staff are being utilized efficiently with respect to patient load. Optimal capacity is often evidenced by reasonable waiting times, defined as approximately 20 minutes, before being seen by a provider. At optimal capacity, the reimbursement for the patient at least covers and more often exceeds the cost of the visit. At optimal capacity, the practice can handle additional patient visits without the need to add expenses in the form of staff, physical space, or technology. At optimal capacity, the practice can afford to take contracts based solely on variable costs.

Maximum capacity defines a situation where the practice is figuratively "bursting at the seams," waiting times are significant (longer than 1 hour), it takes weeks or months for a patient to schedule a visit, or staff and providers are typically overworked. In a situation of maximum capacity, the practice is normally understaffed and undersized for the patient visit load, and taking on any new patients or managed care contracts would necessitate the addition of staff, physical space, and new or additional technology. At this point, any new contract will result in costs above and beyond the normal contract cost.

PROJECTING CONTRACT VOLUME

Once utilization-per-thousand calculations have been completed, it is possible to project visit volume as a result of proposed new contracts. In order for this to occur, it is first necessary to know the number of "lives," or insured subscribers, under this contract who will visit the practice for care. To calculate visit rates, invert the calculation for utilization per thousand, as follows:

(Utilization per Thousand * Lives)/1,000

Based on Exhibit 8.4, take a proposed contract that has 1,000 insured lives to be directed to the practice. Using code 10060 as an example, you would multiply the utilization per thousand for that code by the 5,000 insured lives and then divide by 1,000, as follows:

8.29 * 5,000 = 41,450 and 41,450/1,000 = 41.5

In this example, you could estimate that, based on the new contract, you would have an additional 41.5 visits that would be coded as 10060. To determine the total number of visits under the proposed contract, calculate the sum of the Addt'l Freq column.

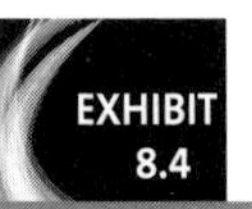

EXHIBIT 8.4 Projections for Patient Visit Volume

Code	Description	Fee	Current Freq	Utilization per Thousand	Addt'l Freq
10060	Drainage of skin abscess	$129	75	8.29	41
17000	Destroy benign/premlg lesion	$146	410	45.34	227
45330	Diagnostic sigmoidoscopy	$243	29	3.21	16
58150	Total hysterectomy	$1432	40	4.42	22
59025	Fetal non-stress test	$137	253	27.98	140
99203	Office/outpatient visit, new	$151	902	99.75	499
99213	Office/outpatient visit, est	$97	15543	1,718.79	8,594
99243	Office consultation	$191	24	2.65	13
	TOTALS		17276	1,910.43	9,552

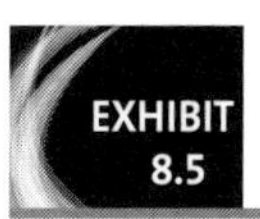

EXHIBIT 8.5 Projecting Contract Cost Using Variable Expenses

Code	Description	Fee	Current Freq	Utilization per Thousand	Addt'l Freq	Variable Cost per Procedure	Cost of New Contract
10060	Drainage of skin abscess	$129	75	8.29	41	$23.22	962.90
17000	Destroy benign/premlg lesion	$146	410	45.34	227	$15.26	3,459.36
45330	Diagnostic sigmoidoscopy	$243	29	3.21	16	$30.35	486.65
58150	Total hysterectomy	$1432	40	4.42	22	$230.38	5,095.21
59025	Fetal non-stress test	$137	253	27.98	140	$10.38	1,452.03
99203	Office/outpatient visit, new	$151	902	99.75	499	$24.18	12,059.25
99213	Office/outpatient visit, est	$97	15543	1,718.79	8,594	$13.28	114,127.52
99243	Office consultation	$191	24	2.65	13	$30.40	403.41
	TOTALS		17276	1,910.43	9,552		138,046.33

PROJECTING CONTRACT COST

Building on the last section, take the calculated additional frequencies to estimate what the cost of the contract will be for the practice. This can be done using either total or variable expenses (or both). The calculation is very straightforward: multiply the projected volume for each code times the cost for each code, as shown in Exhibit 8.5. In this example, variable costs are used to project the cost of the contract. Based upon the calculations used, an additional cost to the practice of $138,046 would be projected.

Much of this assumption of variable expense is based on the practice being at optimal capacity. In an excess capacity situation, you would use the total cost of the contract instead of variable costs. For maximum capacity practices, the cost of adding new staff, technology, and physical space would need to be considered in order to manage the additional 10,000 or so visits, in turn adding these costs back into the contract amount.

Calculation of cost per member per month is effective within the practice entity when using practice-specific data.

CALCULATING PER MEMBER PER MONTH COSTS

When capitation was the rage, most gatekeeper contracts were based on payments calculated as PMPM. This meant that the practice was paid, in advance, a stipend for each insured life within the provider's patient panel. If the practice was able to manage the patient care for less than the stipend, it would be profitable under the contract. But if the costs to care for the patient were more than the stipend, the practice would lose money. One method to determine potential profitability for the contract is to first calculate the PMPM cost for the practice and then compare that to the proposed PMPM rate. To calculate the PMPM costs, divide the total cost per procedure by the number of lives and then divide that product by 12.

In Exhibit 8.6, let's use procedure code 58150 as an example. The total cost for the practice at their utilization-per-thousand rate and the number of active lives is $31,396.40. Divide that by the number of active patients (9,043) and then divide again by 12, as follows:

Capitation, although decreasing in popularity, is still holding its own in some urban markets and particularly in the northwest United States.

$$\$31{,}396.40/9{,}043 = \$3.47 \text{ (approximate cost per active patient)}$$
$$\$3.47/12 = \$0.2893 \text{ (approximate cost per active patient per month)}$$

Exhibit 8.7 uses the same methodology to calculate the variable cost PMPM using the same sample data set.

APPLICATIONS TO CAPITATION

Capitation, although no longer a growing form of managed care in the United States, still has a reasonable market share in many areas. This is especially true in metropolitan areas and in the northwest. Capitation is a method of healthcare provider reimbursement within a managed care system in which a fixed, predetermined amount is paid to the provider for each person enrolled or assigned to the provider for a given period. This is

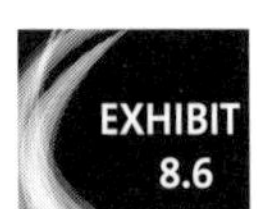
EXHIBIT 8.6

Total Per Member Per Month Costs

Code	Description	Fee	Current Freq	Utilization per Thousand	Cost per Procedure	Total Cost per Procedure	Cost PMPM
10060	Drainage of skin abscess	$129	75	8.29	$79.12	$5,934.00	$0.055
17000	Destroy benign/premlg lesion	$146	410	45.34	$51.99	$21,315.90	$0.196
45330	Diagnostic sigmoidoscopy	$243	29	3.21	$103.39	$2,998.31	$0.028
58150	Total hysterectomy	$1432	40	4.42	$784.91	$31,396.40	$0.289
59025	Fetal non-stress test	$137	253	27.98	$35.35	$8,943.55	$0.082
99203	Office/outpatient visit, new	$151	902	99.75	$82.38	$74,306.76	$0.685
99213	Office/outpatient visit, est	$97	15543	1,718.79	$45.26	$703,476.18	$6.483
99243	Office consultation	$191	24	2.65	$103.57	$2,485.68	$0.023
	TOTALS		17276			$850,856.78	$7.841

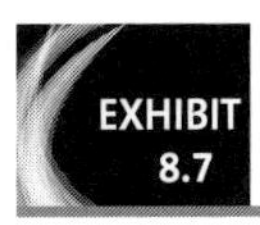

EXHIBIT 8.7

Variable Per Member Per Month Costs

Code	Description	Fee	Current Freq	Utilization per Thousand	Variable Cost per Procedure	Total Cost per Procedure	Variable Cost PMPM
10060	Drainage of skin abscess	$129	75	8.29	$23.22	$1,741.72	$0.016
17000	Destroy benign/premlg lesion	$146	410	45.34	$15.26	$6,256.54	$0.058
45330	Diagnostic sigmoidoscopy	$243	29	3.21	$30.35	$880.05	$0.008
58150	Total hysterectomy	$1432	40	4.42	$230.38	$9,215.33	$0.085
59025	Fetal non-stress test	$137	253	27.98	$10.38	$2,625.07	$0.024
99203	Office/outpatient visit, new	$151	902	99.75	$24.18	$21,810.18	$0.201
99213	Office/outpatient visit, est	$97	15543	1,718.79	$13.28	$206,481.06	$1.903
99243	Office consultation	$191	24	2.65	$30.40	$729.59	$0.007
	TOTALS		17276			$249,739.53	$2.301

without regard to the actual number or nature of services provided to these enrollees.

For example, a family practice has signed up with a plan and has 300 people select it as their primary care provider. The practice is paid $12.00 PMPM for all services. This equals a monthly payment to the practice of $3,600.

When working in a capitation environment, filling beds in a hospital is no longer important because profitability is often tied to managing the care of the patient. Medical groups begin to focus more on service prevention, which could be quite costly. Under a fee-for-service plan, utilization of costly diagnostic and surgical procedures would produce a profit; under capitation, these procedures could dilute the profitability for the practice. If managed properly, some practices may benefit because there are no receivables and, in rare cases, the practice may receive a bonus based upon utilization performance.

Capitation presents a paradigm shift from the fee-for-service mentality. Where procedures once generated revenue, they now contribute to financial liability.

Because capitation is the product of usage of service (i.e., utilization) of service times the cost for each service per member (i.e., person) for a given time period, there are inherent risks to this type of arrangement. Following are the most common risks the practice should be aware of and be able to assess for each capitation-based contract:

- *Price risk:* Is the market value below the practice's cost of doing business?
- *Utilization risk:* Could the enrollees' utilization end up being too high?

- *Market risk:* The health maintenance organization (HMO) may have to reduce its premiums in order to maintain or gain market share. This usually reduces the availability of funds for healthcare providers (i.e., the capitation premium may get cut).
- *Selection risk:* Are the people who choose the practice or are referred to the practice for care sicker or more expensive to treat?
- *Partner risk:* To be successful in a capitated environment, other providers, the insurer, and the purchasers involved in the plan must do their parts.
- *Regulatory risk:* Government regulation could impact the spending of funds for healthcare services. For example, the government could reduce the amount it pays to HMOs to cover Medicare patients enrolled in a senior capitated plan. This in turn reduces funds available to the healthcare providers.

Utilization-per-thousand data are only applicable to the patient population from which the data were taken. Age and sex of the population control the utilization-per-thousand ratios.

Socioeconomics of Utilization

To this point, you have calculated utilization values based on the practice's own experience with its own patients. Even in projecting visit levels and costs, it was assumed that the patient population being proposed under the contract has characteristics that are similar to those of patients currently being seen. The greatest variables for calculating utilization per thousand are age and sex. Older and younger populations consume more healthcare services than those who are middle-aged. Women consume more healthcare services than men. Socioeconomic demographics can also play a big role because those in lower socioeconomic categories tend to consume more healthcare resources than those in other categories.

When considering a large capitation contract, it is important to assess the characteristics of the population that is insured under the contract. If the value (or risk) of the contract is sizeable, it is highly recommended that the practice contract an actuary to evaluate the age/sex demographics in order to normalize the utilization distribution calculations to those population characteristics. One saying that holds true is this, if you can't afford an actuary, you can't afford the contract.

Evaluating the Rate

First, you must determine the underlying assumptions of the proposed capitated rate. The assumptions could include, for example, the demographic mix and how age and sex are built into the rate. By analyzing this information, you can determine whether or not the assumptions for the physician's service area are accurate. For example, an assumption could be that the population within a service area is composed mainly of young patients, when in fact the service area has been aging quite a bit over the past few years.

If the financial commitment to the contract is substantial, consider hiring an actuary who has experience with capitation. It's not cheap, but neither is a bad capitation contract.

When evaluating the physician's proposed capitation rate, you must determine whether it is an aggregate rate or is broken down into age/sex cell categories. Always attempt to negotiate a rate based on age/sex categories because an insured population is never constant. Men and women of different ages move in and out of the HMO plan. If the physician's capitated payment is based on an aggregate rate and older (i.e., more costly) people enroll in the plan, the physician will not be compensated adequately. The physician's capitated payments should be adjusted as different types of people enroll in and leave the plan. The HMO should be able to provide the practice with a breakdown of the age/sex cell categories with corresponding capitation rates for each category. Also make sure the funds available for capitation payments are not based on a "percent of premium." Try to avoid this whenever possible. In this situation, a percent of the premiums received by the HMO is designated for certain provider categories (i.e., for all medical services). If the HMO has to lower premium rates in order to compete in the marketplace, the providers in turn will receive less money.

As stated earlier, when in doubt, engage the services of an actuary to assist in the evaluation of the proposed capitation rate. Make sure the actuary has healthcare experience and be sure to ask for his or her fee structure. Hiring an outside actuary will not be cheap.

Calculating Visit and Cost Potential

When the calculation of visit and cost potential was discussed previously, you were using data from the practice. Now, you need to consider using a data set from outside the practice because it may be more applicable to the population's characteristics. The HMO should be able to provide the practice with the utilization-per-thousand data they use to calculate payment. If they are unable (or most often, unwilling) to provide this data set, it can be obtained from a third-party. In a worst-case scenario, use internal data.

The following is typical methodology for calculating a capitation contract (Exhibit 8.8):

1. Know your fee and frequency for each procedure code.
2. Obtain RVU and geographic adjustment factor components (if using the RBRVS).
3. Obtain the total number of covered lives from the HMO or carrier.
4. Use cost accounting data to determine your cost for performing each procedure.
5. Obtain the projected annual utilization per 1,000 members. This can be done using the data from the HMO source, hiring an actuary, or purchasing third-party actuarial data.
6. Calculate the cost per member per month. This is done by multiplying the cost per procedure by utilization per 1,000 members. Then divide by 1,000 to get the cost per member then dividing by 12 to get the cost per member per month.
7. Calculate annual projected utilization. This is done by taking the utilization per thousand, dividing by 1,000, and then multiplying by the number of covered lives (8,000).
8. Calculate the annual contract cost by multiplying the utilization by the procedure cost.

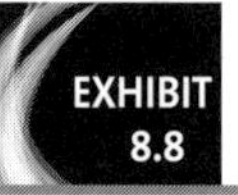

Sample Capitation Contract Cost and Visit Analysis

Code	RVU TOT	Cost	HMO Util/1000	PMPM	Utilization	Contract
10060	1.60	$11.23	28.447	0.027	227.58	2556
10061	3.18	$22.32	1.789	0.003	14.31	319
10120	1.70	$11.93	3.936	0.004	31.49	376
10121	3.76	$26.39	8.051	0.018	64.41	1700
10140	2.01	$14.10	23.796	0.028	190.36	2686
10160	1.58	$11.09	7.693	0.007	61.55	683
11000	1.35	$9.47	1.073	0.001	8.59	81
11040	0.94	$6.59	18.965	0.010	151.72	1001
11042	1.85	$12.98	0.179	0.000	1.43	19
11050	0.83	$5.82	7.157	0.003	57.25	334
11051	1.21	$8.49	0.358	0.000	2.86	24
11052	1.31	$9.19	0.179	0.000	1.43	13
11420	1.58	$11.09	9.840	0.009	78.72	873
Cost per unit:		$7.02		0.841	3,871.70	80760

► Using Standard Deviation Models

One of the biggest problems in developing capitation models is the assumption of validity and the accuracy of the utilization-per-thousand data. In most instances, unless a competent actuary has been contracted to develop these numbers, utilization-per-thousand data should be very suspect. This is unfortunate because the entire cost analysis is based upon these data. In order to develop a risk analysis or best-case/worst-case scenarios, the entire analysis should be run using reasonable variants of the utilization-per-thousand data set. This can be done by using standard deviation amounts or by developing your own variables. Using standard z-table distributions, which standardize the distance from the mean for a normal distribution, you would calculate the utilization-per-thousand data using 1 standard deviation (+/–34.1 percent), 2 standard deviations (+/–47.7 percent), or 3 standard deviations (+/–49.9 percent). Using 3 standard deviations, you would be confident that the utilization-per-thousand scenarios you develop would occur within the plus/minus range 98.8 percent of the time. In this manner, you would be able to calculate the potential risk within a safe limit.

Building best-case and worst-case scenarios may help you to see the big picture as it pertains to both the potential for profitability and risk assessment.

Exhibits 8.9 and 8.10 are example capitation worksheets that illustrate the differences in PMPM costs, utilization expectations, and total contract

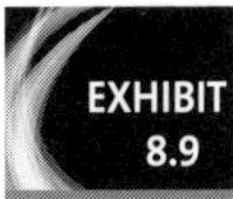
EXHIBIT 8.9

Utilization Calculations Using the Mean –3 Standard Deviation

Code	RVU TOT	Cost	Util/1000	PMPM	Utilization	Contract
10060	1.60	$11.23	14.252	0.013	114.02	1280
10061	3.18	$22.32	0.896	0.002	7.17	160
10120	1.70	$11.93	1.972	0.002	15.78	188
10121	3.76	$26.39	4.034	0.009	32.27	852
10140	2.01	$14.10	11.922	0.014	95.37	1346
10160	1.58	$11.09	3.854	0.004	30.83	342
11000	1.35	$9.47	0.538	0.000	4.30	41
11040	0.94	$6.59	9.501	0.005	76.01	502
11042	1.85	$12.98	0.090	0.000	0.72	9
11050	0.83	$5.82	3.585	0.002	28.68	167
11051	1.21	$8.49	0.179	0.000	1.43	12
11052	1.31	$9.19	0.090	0.000	0.72	7
11420	1.58	$11.09	4.930	0.005	39.44	437
Cost per unit:		$7.02		0.421	1,939.72	40461

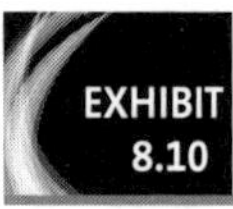

EXHIBIT 8.10

Utilization Calculations Using the Mean +3 Standard Deviation

Code	RVU TOT	Cost	Util/1000	PMPM	Utilization	Contract
10060	1.60	$11.23	42.643	0.040	341.14	3831
10061	3.18	$22.32	2.682	0.005	21.46	479
10120	1.70	$11.93	5.900	0.006	47.20	563
10121	3.76	$26.39	12.069	0.027	96.55	2548
10140	2.01	$14.10	35.670	0.042	285.36	4026
10160	1.58	$11.09	11.532	0.011	92.26	1023
11000	1.35	$9.47	1.609	0.001	12.87	122
11040	0.94	$6.59	28.428	0.016	227.43	1501
11042	1.85	$12.98	0.268	0.000	2.15	28
11050	0.83	$5.82	10.728	0.005	85.82	500
11051	1.21	$8.49	0.536	0.000	4.29	36
11052	1.31	$9.19	0.268	0.000	2.15	20
Cost per unit:		$7.02		1.261	5803.68	121060

costs by deviating from the mean by –3 standard deviations and +3 standard deviations.

You can see a significant variance between all three levels of utilization-per-thousand numbers. For example, if the HMO were to offer the practice $1.33 PMPM to manage the subscriber base, it would appear that there would be a profit to be made of almost $0.20 PMPM. This, of course, assumes that the mean utilization-per-thousand numbers are accurate. Based upon a best-case scenario (mean –3 standard deviations), the practice would stand to profit a little more than $0.76 PMPM. Based upon a worst-case scenario, however, the practice risks a loss of $0.37 PMPM. Based upon total utilization levels, this could be a significant financial loss to the practice over the entire contract.

In the latter worse-case scenario, the practice could propose a shared risk agreement with the HMO whereby the HMO would contribute up to 50 percent of any loss that occurred as a result of the utilization-per-thousand numbers being higher than the mean projection. For example, if utilization did turn out to be as high as +3 standard deviations, then the insurance company would pay an additional $0.185 PMPM, half of the $0.37 amount lost under the contract. In some cases, the HMO will agree to this on the condition that the practice shares 50 percent of the

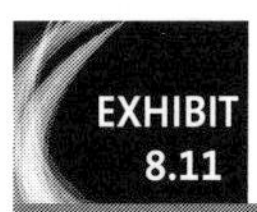

Exhibit 8.11 Standard Deviation Risk Analysis

	PMPM Costs	Utilization Amounts	Contract Cost
Mean Minus 3 STD	$0.568	1,939.72	$54,546
Mean	$1.134	3,871.70	$108,874
Mean Plus 3 STD	$1.700	5,803.68	$163,202

difference between the projected mean utilization per thousand and the actual utilization per thousand if it is less than the mean. Again, for this example, if the actual utilization per thousand was at the –3 standard deviation level, the practice would pay $0.38 PMPM back to the HMO or half of the profit amount under the contract (Exhibit 8.11).

In many cases, however, it is most likely that the practice will not be able to negotiate a rate with the HMO; therefore, the comparisons should be used to calculate relative risk. The practice should assess the worst-case scenario from an overall financial standpoint balanced against the potential risk of loss if the contract is not accepted.

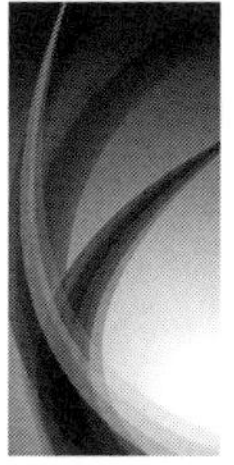

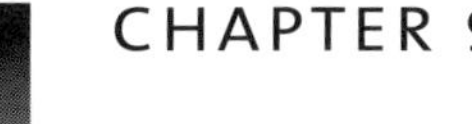

CHAPTER 9

Compliance Risk Assessment

The medical practitioner in the United States is oriented toward providing quality care. It's engrained within the educational process and, for most, simply a part of the cultural paradigm. The payer, on the other hand, is oriented toward profit, and this creates a natural conflict of interest between what should be business partners. The physician provides quality service and expects to get paid and the payer does what it can to not pay for those services. And even when payment is made, the payer comes back in an attempt to reclaim what was never theirs in the first place, that is, the payment for services rendered.

In any industry, except healthcare, business is transacted based on an exchange of products or services for some equivalent value, such as money. It's a law, so to speak. If, after engaging in a transaction, the buyer discovers that the product or service was not as represented or the buyer pays for a product or service but does not receive what he or she paid for, the buyer has a right to have the purchase amount mitigated through either a reduction in price or a refund. Should it be different in healthcare? Not necessarily. If a practice bills for a service that is not provided, they should have to pay back the money. If a practitioner misrepresents a procedure or service being provided, then some adjustment should be made. If, however, the practice bills for a service that, in good faith, was provided to a patient, the amount for the service should not only be paid but the practice should be allowed to keep the money.

In today's practice environment, there seems to be a "feeding frenzy" by both government and private payers to either *not* pay for services provided to a patient by his or her physician or to come back later and demand repayment. And although this is not a book on auditing, the resource-based relative value scale (RBRVS) can, in fact, play an important role in helping the practice conduct a compliance risk assessment.

THE AUDIT EVENT

An audit normally takes place for one of three reasons. It is a:

- Random event
- Qui-Tam event
- Benchmarking event

I once knew a pathologist who spent two years defending an Office of the Inspector General audit. He said that it was like having an autopsy without the benefit of death.

There are times when an audit may be random; you just happen to be in the wrong place at the wrong time. Perhaps the auditing agency is required to audit a certain number of practices within a given geographic area and, voilà, there you are. As seen in the Comprehensive Error Rate Testing study, some carriers have a higher rate of improper payment than others, which could subject practices in those geographic areas to a higher rate of random audit and review.

A Qui-Tam event occurs when someone, that is, a whistle-blower, reports an aberrant practice. In fact, some of the biggest audit cases I've seen have been in response to whistle-blowers. A February 23, 2012, article in *USA Today*, titled "Whistle-blowers key in healthcare fraud fight," revealed that the federal government brought in more than $2 billion in whistle-blower settlements and judgments.

A benchmarking event is likely responsible for the highest ratio of auditing events for medical practices. Quite simply, if what you are doing differs significantly from what your peers are doing, then you are increasing the probability that you will become the target of an audit.

THE AUDIT PROCESS

There are four primary phases within the audit process:

1. Pre-audit risk assessment
2. Intra-audit qualitative review
3. Post-audit analysis
4. Appeals process

An understanding of each phase is critical in order to mitigate any damage that may result from an audit of your practice.

The pre-audit risk assessment phase requires that the practice take a step back and look at the practice the way that an outsider (or an auditor) would. For example, pretend that you are an auditor. When you look at your practice, what do you see? Do you see a well-run and well-managed entity with regard to coding and billing or do you see a gold mine for recovering payments? This is done by conducting a procedure code, modifier, and evaluation and management utilization analysis of the practice.

The intra-audit qualitative review is, in effect, the chart audit. This often becomes a battle of the experts in that the practice confirms the validity of the codes used and supports medical necessity while the auditor argues the opposite. This is, perhaps, the toughest phase and consumes significant resources as the practice goes through the appeals process.

The resource-based relative value scale database is commonly referred to by auditors. Why? Because relative value units translate into dollars and they can be used as a proxy to estimate the impact of an extrapolation audit.

Phase 3 involves a more statistically oriented approach, such as determining whether what the auditor calls a random sample is truly a statistically valid random sample. Or whether the correct measurements of location were used and, in the case of an extrapolation audit, whether the proper extrapolation techniques and calculations were used.

The appeals phase relies upon the pre-, intra-, and post-audit analyses, and success is dependent upon the thoroughness of your work.

Having said all of this, it is the first phase where RBRVS can be the most effective and, as such, is what this chapter is about. By now, you should have an understanding of the relationships between relative value units (RVUs) and resource consumption and between RVUs and money. From the government's perspective, each RVU is worth a given amount in dollars based on the Centers for Medicare & Medicaid Services (CMS)-assigned conversion factor. For private payers that base their fee schedules on RBRVS or Medicare, the implications are about the same. So if you accept that these relationships are factual, then you can proceed to look at the variance in RVU values from the perspective of procedure code utilization to view your risk in the same way that the auditor views opportunity.

PROCEDURE CODE UTILIZATION

The process begins by benchmarking utilization of your procedures codes against some standard or control group. Here data obtained from the Physician/Supplier Procedure Summary Master File (P/SPSMF), which contains 100 percent of all Medicare claims filed during any given period, is used. To be sure, some will argue that this is not the best of benchmarks because utilization of services and procedures by Medicare patients does not necessarily represent that for non-Medicare patients. This is not an entirely unfounded concern. Actuarially speaking, age and sex are two of the most important predictors when regressing utilization of medical services and procedures. However, because the database is large (more than 2.5 billion lines) and readily available (can be purchased for $250 or obtained as the Part-B Extract Summary System data set for free on the CMS Web site), the relatively small error is acceptable for most folks. More importantly, this tends to be the same database that government auditors depend on when looking for benchmark-stimulated audit events. So even though it may not be perfect, it definitely provides a high degree of value.

► Data Requirements

In order to conduct the procedure code utilization, you need to be able to produce a readable electronic file that contains at least the following information:

- Provider name or ID
- Procedure code
- RVU value
- Frequency

The file might look something like Exhibit 9.1.

You can aggregate the data any way you want; however, the least granular data needs to be specialty specific. For example, if you are a single-specialty practice, you can aggregate the frequency data for the practice. If you are a multispecialty practice, you must aggregate at least by the individual specialties. It is recommended that you follow the above example and aggregate by provider because it only takes one provider to stimulate an audit and it provides the most efficient method for assessing specific risk.

The next item you will need is the comparison file, which is available through some commercial vendors as well as the CMS Web site. This file contains the top 10 procedure codes reported by 70 different specialties and allows you to benchmark your data, testing it for variability and significance.

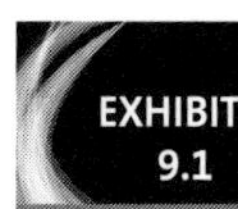

EXHIBIT 9.1

Procedure Code Data by Provider

Provider ID	Procedure Code	Freq	RVU	Total RVUs
N002	25000	16	8.82	141.12
N001	27130	26	38.19	999.94
D001	27236	14	21.70	303.74
H001	27506	4	35.22	140.88
H001	28262	4	35.30	141.20
D001	29880	12	11.78	141.41
F001	29888	40	26.05	1,042.00
M001	76000	114	2.68	305.52
M002	99202	166	1.86	308.76
N002	99203	110	2.71	298.10
O003	99214	374	2.71	1,013.54
O003	99231	288	1.05	302.40

A friend once told me that it's not how you feel but how you look that's important. This is very true when it comes to how your utilization compares to that of your peers. If you are way off, can you explain why?

Conducting the Analysis

As stated, comparisons are made against some peer-based control group. Here the P/SPS national database is used. Critically, the top 10 to 25 codes should be considered for comparison; however, you can calculate the number of procedure codes that make up the top 80 percent and use those. Because you are basing your assessment on RVU values, you may want to take the top 10 to 25 codes based on the total RVUs, sorted in descending order. For example, your data set may look like that in Exhibit 9.2.

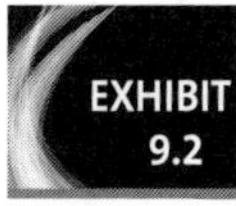

EXHIBIT 9.2

Relative Value Units in Descending Order

Procedure Code	Freq	Total RVUs
99213	5,868	10,194.48
99243	1,712	5,688.29
99242	1,616	3,923.97
27130	96	3,471.97
27447	84	3,248.67
20610	1,674	3,133.23
99214	1,116	2,908.07
99203	1,072	2,778.52
27130	70	2,531.64
64721	220	2,252.40

9.3 Relative Value Units in Descending Order

Orthopedic Surgery

CPT Code	Description	Work RVUs	National		Practice		Total RVUs
			Rank	Percent	Rank	Percent	
27447	Total knee arthroplasty	23.25	1	10.20%	3	4.92%	3,949
99213	Office/outpatient visit, est	0.97	2	8.28%	1	8.24%	6,614
20610	Drain/inject. joint/bursa	0.79	3	6.62%	6	3.82%	3,062
99214	Office/outpatient visit, est	1.50	4	4.00%	10	2.34%	1,875
27130	Total hip arthroplasty	21.79	5	3.98%	5	4.25%	3,410
99203	Office/outpatient visit, new	1.42	6	3.55%	7	2.76%	2,211
99204	Office/outpatient visit, new	2.43	7	2.26%	16	1.51%	1,212
27245	Treat thigh fracture	18.18	8	2.21%			
27236	Treat thigh fracture	17.61	9	1.95%	8	2.59%	2,078
99212	Office/outpatient visit, est	0.48	10	1.63%	23	1.06%	847
22612	Lumbar spine fusion	23.53	11	1.45%			
29827	Arthroscop rotator cuff repr	15.59	12	1.23%	14	1.63%	1,312
29826	Shoulder arthroscopy/surgery	9.16	13	1.22%	15	1.60%	1,284
29881	Knee arthroscopy/surgery	8.71	14	1.13%	11	2.33%	1,867
97110	Therapeutic exercises	0.45	15	1.11%			
63047	Removal of spinal lamina	15.37	16	0.96%			
29880	Knee arthroscopy/surgery	9.45	17	0.95%	25	0.88%	704
23472	Reconstruct shoulder joint	22.65	18	0.87%			
73721	Mri jnt of lwr extre w/o dye	1.35	19	0.81%			
73562	X-ray exam of knee, 3	0.18	20	0.81%			
64721	Carpal tunnel surgery	4.97	21	0.74%	24	0.95%	760
73560	X-ray exam of knee, 1 or 2	0.17	22	0.70%			
27244	Treat thigh fracture	18.18	23	0.66%			
20680	Removal of support implant	5.96	24	0.63%	18	1.43%	1,145
73510	X-ray exam of hip	0.21	25	0.60%			

The next step is to create a comparison table. Exhibit 9.3 provides a comparison of the top 25 procedures reported from the P/SPS file for this specialty by the frequency reported for the practice for the same specialty.

Now take a look at the first entry: procedure code 27447. For all orthopedic surgeons, 27447 accounts for the highest RVU value reported, ranked number 1 and reported as 10.20 percent of all RVUs. For the practice, it is reported as number 3, accounting for 4.92 percent, or about half of what its peer group reports. Now take a look at code 29881.

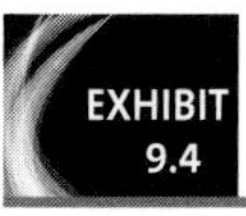

Expected Utilization vs. Observed Utilization

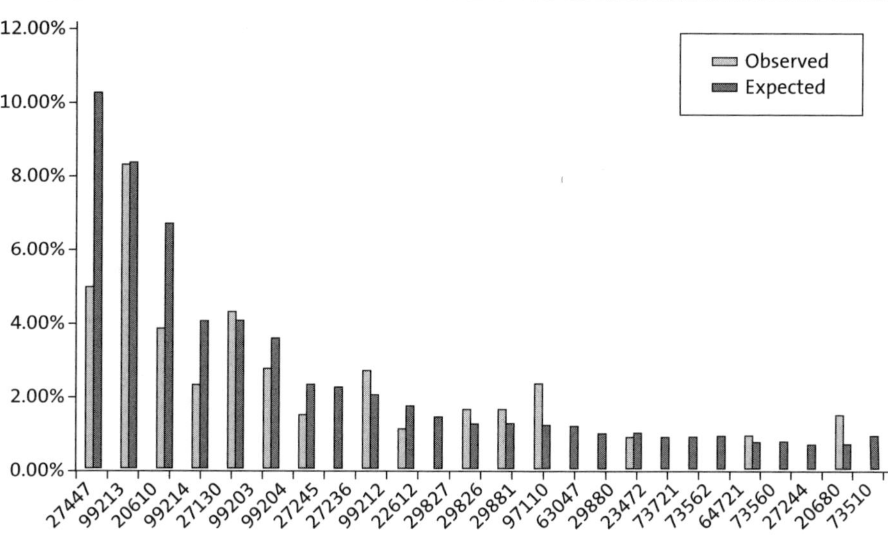

Nationally, this code is reported as number 14 in rank order, accounting for 1.13 percent of all RVUs reported. For the practice, it is ranked number 11 but reports just over twice as many RVUs as a percent of all RVUs for the practice. This provides a target for the auditor because RVUs translate to dollars and the greater your variance (in excess), the more dollar signs the auditor sees.

It is suggested that you conduct a statistical test, or a chi-square test, on your comparisons. This provides homogeneity, which, in simple terms, measures how alike one data set is to another. Exhibit 9.4 is commonly referred to as a chi-square graph. As you can see, it makes it much easier to identify the difference between your data and the control group. For example, for the first set of bars (code 27447), you can clearly see that fewer RVUs were observed than expected while for code 29881, more RVUs were reported than expected. And remember, "expected" refers to the comparison (or control) group.

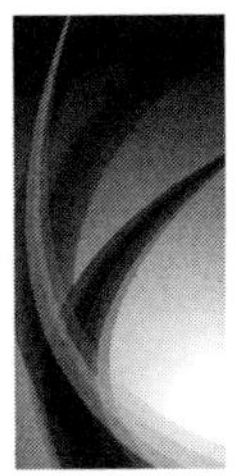

Glossary

Adjusted charges

Adjusted charges are the total amounts expected to be paid by patients or third-party payers. These figures can be calculated by taking gross charges and subtracting the adjustments from third-party payers and charge restrictions from Medicare/Medicaid.

American Medical Association (AMA)

Established in 1847, the American Medical Association (AMA) is the largest association of medical doctors in the United States. It promotes professionalism in medicine and sets standards for medical education, practice, and ethics. Learn more about the AMA by visiting its Web site at www.ama-assn.org.

Benchmarking

Benchmarking is the ongoing process of establishing a standard of excellence and comparing activities to that standard, whether it is internal or external to the organization.

Centers for Medicare & Medicaid Services (CMS)

The Centers for Medicare & Medicaid Services (CMS) is a federal agency within the U.S. Department of Health and Human Services. CMS runs the Medicare and the Medicaid programs — two national health care programs that benefit more than 75 million Americans. Together with the Health Resources and Services Administration, CMS also runs the State Children's Health Insurance Program (SCHIP), a program that is expected to cover many of the approximately 10 million uninsured children in the United States. CMS was formerly known as the Health Care Financing Administration (HCFA).

Code ranges

A code range is a group of codes that encompass related procedures or services. Examples of ranges include surgery codes 10040 to 69990, evaluation and management (E/M) codes 99201 to 99499, and medicine codes 90281 to 99199. The logic behind this basic categorization is that charges and RVUs tend to be similar within the same range of codes. Naturally, the code ranges would have to be much smaller than these broad categories in order for this logic to bear itself out.

Conversion factor

A conversion factor is the dollar amount paid per RVU by third-party payers. It converts RVUs into money for reimbursement of medical procedures.

Cost-based fee schedule

A cost-based fee schedule is based on the actual cost the practice incurs to provide the service or procedure to the patient. The cost for each procedure is determined, and a percentage is added on top of it to act as a buffer against discounts and bad debts. The "cost-plus" amount then becomes the practice's standard fee for that procedure.

Current Procedural Terminology (CPT) codes

Current Procedural Terminology (CPT) codes are copyrighted and have been maintained by the AMA since 1966. CPTs are unique, five-character billing codes for medical procedures, providing an accurate, uniform language that describes medical, surgical, and diagnostic services. These codes serve as an effective means for reliable, nationwide communication among physicians, other health care providers, patients, and various third parties.

Direct expenses

Direct expenses are costs that can be linked to or incurred by a specific individual (for example, automobiles, cellular phones, medical conferences, travel, meals, and entertainment).

Fee-for-service (FFS) charges

Fee-for-service (FFS) charges are gross charges at the practice's established, undiscounted rates.

Fee schedule

A fee schedule is a list of the practice's standard rates for providing procedures and services to patients. The three main types of fee schedules are historical- based, market-based, and cost-based.

Full-time equivalent (FTE)

According to MGMA, a full-time equivalent (FTE) physician or non-physician provider works at least the number of hours the practice considers to be the minimum for a normal work week, which could be 37.5, 40, 50, or some other standard number of hours.

Geographic Adjustment Factors

CMS uses a single number called Geographic Adjustment Factors (GAFs) to compare one payment locality to another and to show the difference between the adjusted GPCIs per payment locality from one calendar year to the next. In effect, GAFs are a rollup of adjusted GPCIs.

Geographic Practice Cost Indices (GPCIs)

Geographic Practice Cost Indices (GPCIs) are adjustment factors created by CMS to account for the geographic cost differences across the United States. These factors are used to calculate Medicare reimbursements when multiplied by the RVUs associated with each CPT-4 code. GPCIs are divided into the same three components as the RVUs within the RBRVS: physician work, practice expense, and malpractice.

Gross charges

Gross charges are the full dollar value, at the practice's established undiscounted rates, of services provided to all patients, before reduction by charitable adjustments, professional courtesy adjustments, contractual adjustments, employee discounts, bad debts, and so on. For both Medicare participating and nonparticipating providers, gross charges should include the practice's full undiscounted charge and not the Medicare limiting charge.

HCFA's Common Procedure Coding System (HCPCS)

HCFA's Common Procedure Coding System (HCPCS) is a standardized method or system for reporting professional services, procedures, and supplies. HCPCS are typically paid on a flat rate and, therefore, do not have RVUs assigned to the codes because none of them are required to calculate a reimbursement rate. Even though HCFA changed its name to CMS in 2001, as of this writing HCPCS has not yet followed suit.

Health Care Financing Administration (HCFA)

The Health Care Financing Administration (HCFA) changed to CMS in 2001. See CMS for further information.

Cost per mRVU

The cost per malpractice RVU is calculated by dividing the total malpractice premium expense by the total malpractice RVUs. This indicates the cost of malpractice coverage per RVU.

Cost per peRVU

The cost per practice expense RVU is calculated by dividing the total practice expenses by the sum of the total practice expense RVUs. This should be monitored as an indicator for cost vs. volume.

Cost per wRVU

The cost per work RVU is calculated by dividing the sum of the total provider compensation by the total work RVUs. This is an indication of what a practice is, on average, paying their providers per work RVU.

RVUs per FTE

The RVUs per FTE indicator is the average number of RVUs produced per FTE provider during a specific time period. It is calculated by dividing the total number of RVUs produced by the total FTE count. This indicator can be a good productivity measure by which to compare providers within a specialty.

RVUs per procedure

The RVUs per procedure indicator is the average amount of RVUs produced during each procedure. It is calculated by dividing the total number of RVUs produced by the number of procedures completed. This can be a good indica- tor for both procedure and patient complexity.

wRVUs per FTE

The average number of wRVUs accumulated during the given time period assuming a 1.0 FTE status for the provider.

Managed care

Managed care is a broad term that refers to a large variety of reimbursement plans in which third-party payers attempt to control costs by limiting the utilization of medical services, in contrast to the hands-off style of traditional fee-for-service payments.

Managed care fee schedule

A managed care fee schedule is one in which a third-party payer offers the practice a predetermined fee schedule for specific services.

Managed care organization (MCO)

Managed care organization (MCO) is a broad term for managed care health plans, which include health maintenance organizations (HMOs) and preferred provider organizations (PPOs).

MGMA–ACMPE

Since 1926, the association has delivered networking, professional education and resources, political advocacy, and certification for medical practice professionals. The association represents 22,500 members who lead 13,200 organizations nationwide in which some 280,000 physicians provide more than 40 percent of the healthcare services delivered in the United States.

Medicare Physician Fee Schedule (MPFS)

The Medicare Physician Fee Schedule (MPFS) is CMS's reimbursement schedule for physician services rendered to Medicare patients.

Modifiers

Modifiers are used, among other things, to adjust the reimbursement of a service or procedure to account for assistant surgeons, multiple procedures, bilateral procedures, and other factors. If the reimbursement is adjusted for a CPT code, it is logical that the charge and associated RVUs would be similarly affected. Most medical procedure modifiers (with the primary exception of anesthesia codes) make adjustments by percentages rather than amounts.

Nonphysician providers (NPP)

Also referred to as midlevel providers, these providers are specially trained and licensed individuals, employed or contracted, who can provide medical care and billable services. Examples of nonphysician providers include the following:

- Audiologist;
- Certified Registered
- Nurse Anesthetist
- Dietician/nutritionist;
- Midwife;
- Nurse practitioner;
- Occupational therapist;
- Optometrist;
- Perfusionist (surgical);
- Physical therapist;
- Physician assistant (primary care, nonsurgical, or surgical);
- Psychologist;
- Social worker;
- Speech therapist; and
- Surgeon's assistant.

Professional component

The professional component comprises fees paid to the physician for provision of services. When combined, the professional and technical components of a service are referred to as global service.

Relative Value Scale Update Committee (RUC)

The RVS Update Committee (RUC) is a standing committee formed in 1991 that represents all the major medical specialties. It meets on a regular basis throughout each year to review the RVUs assigned to CPT-4 codes and make recommendations to CMS for revisions.

Relative value units (RVUs)

Relative value units (RVUs) are nonmonetary, relative units of measure that indicate the value of health care services and relative differences in resources consumed when providing different procedures and services. RVUs assign relative values or weights to medical procedures primarily for the purpose of reimbursement of services performed. They are used as a standardized method of analyzing resources involved in the provision of services or procedures.

mRVU

The malpractice component of the total RVU is denoted as mRVU. This component measures the risk involved in providing a service.

peRVU

The practice expense component of the total RVU is denoted as peRVU. This component measures the amount of resources attributed to overhead required to provide the service. This includes, but is not limited to, ancillary staff's time and effort and the use of supplies and equipment.

wRVU

The physician work component of the total RVU is denoted as wRVU. This component is designed to measure a provider's skill, effort, and degree of decision-making complexity required for performing a procedure.

tRVU

The total RVUs are denoted as tRVU. It is a sum of the three RVU components: mRVU, peRVU, and wRVU.

Resource-Based Relative Value Scale (RBRVS)

The Resource-Based Relative Value Scale (RBRVS) is the federal government- mandated relative value system implemented in January 1992, used to calculate reimbursement to physicians for medical services provided to Medicare patients. Updated annually, the primary components of the scale include more than 10,000 CPT-4 codes and descriptions, and relative value units for physician work, practice expense, and malpractice assigned to each code.

Technical component

The technical component relates to facilities, equipment, and technical staff required for the delivery of those services. When combined, the "professional and technical" components of a service are referred to as global service.

Usual, customary, and reasonable (UCR)

Usual, customary, and reasonable (UCR) charges were the traditional fee-for- service rates and the universally accepted method of reimbursement until the advent of managed care, the RBRVS, and RVUs. UCR charges are also referred to as customary, prevailing, and reasonable (CPR) charges.

Variable Expenses

Variables expenses are costs that vary in direct proportion to patient volume.

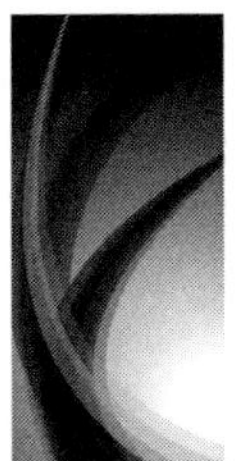

Index

Note: ex. indicates exhibit.

G

H

S

T

U

V

W

Z

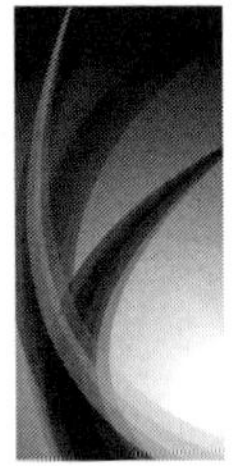

About the Author

Frank Cohen, MBB, MPA, is principal and senior analyst for The Frank Cohen Group, LLC, and a certified Master Black Belt in Lean Six Sigma. As a consultant and researcher, his areas of expertise include data mining, predictive analytics, applied statistics, process improvement, and evidence-based decision support. Cohen is the author of several books and has participated in and published numerous articles and studies. He has trained thousands of physicians, administrators, CPAs, and other healthcare professionals in all areas of healthcare analytics. His experience includes eight years as a physician's assistant in the Navy and as a civilian, clinic administrator, and hospital CEO. His clients include hospitals, large and small medical practices, medical and professional associations, legal and accounting professionals, government agencies, and other healthcare professionals.